LET'S GET THE FEAR OUT OF CANCER

LET'S GET THE FEAR OUT OF CANCER

A holistic approach to illness and to life

Vernon Templemore

Gateway Books, Bath

First published in 1991
by GATEWAY BOOKS
The Hollies, Wellow,
Bath, BA2 8QJ

Set in 10½/12½ pt Palatino by
Ann Buchan (Typesetters), Middlesex
Printed and bound by Billings of Worcester
Cover design by John Douet

British Library Cataloguing in Publication Data:
Templemore, Vernon, 1927–
Let's get the fear out of cancer
1. Cancer
I. Title
158

ISBN 0-946551-00-0

Contents

1

What is Illness?

We often seem to think that illness occurs by chance; it is bad luck, or fate, and we have done nothing to deserve it. 'Why me?' some cancer patients ask. Cancer in particular seems to creep up on us unawares and, although we read that maybe one in three people will get cancer at some time in their lives, somehow it is not going to happen to us. When it does, it can feel like a death sentence. Above all it is the sense of impotence many patients feel when they are faced by the knowledge that they have cancer that is so frightening. They almost certainly know of others who have died of cancer. They believe that they are completely in the hands of the doctors and that there is nothing they can do to help themselves. They hear stories about how stressful the orthodox treatment for cancer can sometimes be and they know that, despite the fact that they are going to have this treatment, there is still no guarantee that they will survive. Orthodox medicine may have made great strides over the past years and more people may be surviving, but far too many still seem to die. The sense of helplessness, when faced by this terrifying prospect, can be paralysing. Later, after their hospital treatment, they may be told by their doctors to go away and forget that they ever had cancer. This is the last thing they can do and some live in constant fear of a recurrence of their illness.

This situation needs to be changed and it can be changed. We need to get the fear out of cancer. Cancer is a

serious illness, but illness is not difficult to understand
and cancer is not difficult to understand. When we understand the causes of illness, we can see what we have to do
to make ourselves better and we can see how we can
prevent ourselves falling ill again in the future. Far too
many people die of cancer unnecessarily.

Some ill health comes as the result of one catastrophi-
cally stressful event. Maybe we are living next to the
nuclear power station when it blows up, or we are
involved in a plane crash, or a car crash, or we fall down
stairs. These events obviously have immediate physical
effects upon us. The vast majority of illnesses, however,
do not come as the result of one stressful event at one
moment in time, they occur as the result of different forms
of relatively lower levels of stress, which build up over a
period of years, like straw piling up on the camel's back;
eventually the camel's back breaks. The stress can be
physical stress, or mental stress, or spiritual stress. In
serious illness all three types of stress will almost certainly
be involved, in some proportion or other. All stress
undermines the immune system and when the immune
system is undermined sufficiently, we fall ill. An efficiently functioning immune system keeps us healthy.
When our immune system is undermined by stress, it has
difficulty in dealing with germs and viruses. We also have
millions and millions of body cells, which are constantly
renewing themselves. When our immune system is functioning properly, it copes adequately with any cells which
change abnormally, as some almost certainly will from
time to time with such large numbers involved. When our
immune system is undermined by too much stress, cells
can continue to grow in abnormal ways and can start to
proliferate abnormally. The body's systems can also start
to work incorrectly and can eventually break down.

The direct physical stress in our lives comes, obviously
enough, from physical factors imposed upon us, or which
we impose upon ourselves – how healthy were our
parents and forebears; how clean or how polluted is our

environment at work and at home; how clean or how polluted is the food and drink we consume; how supple and well exercised do we maintain our bodies; what physical accidents befall us.

The mental and spiritual stress come from our ability to think, and hence our ability to worry about the actual dangers in our lives, about the dangers we believe to exist in our lives, and about whether God is looking after us or not – all the things we cannot control adequately. Unfortunately this worrying has physical effects upon us. Mental and spiritual stress eventually produce physical change in the body, just as physical stress does.

We do not know how or when our primitive consciousness developed to the point where we began to think. The ancestors of man lived as animals, purely by instinct. Instinct and not thought – because we could not think – told us that the dinosaur was dangerous and that to survive, which was our strongest instinct, we either had to fight the dinosaur, or run away from it – the fight or flight response. When danger appeared, our heart rate and our breathing speeded up, so as to get more blood and oxygen to our muscles; we broke out into a cold sweat to help to disperse the extra heat this caused us; our digestion stopped digesting, so that our body could concentrate on more important matters, maybe our bowels and bladder emptied themselves to lighten the load a bit, and our muscles tightened up, so that we could take immediate action. In brief, the adrenalin started to flow – chemical changes took place in our body and our body was automatically prepared for fight or flight. When we fought, or ran away, the chemicals were used up, the chemical balance was restored in our body and our muscles relaxed again as the danger disappeared.

Today, for us more sophisticated beings, the dinosaur has changed its shape. Music hall comedians would have us believe that it has changed into our mother-in-law, and perhaps for some of us it has. It is rather more likely to be our father or mother, who make too many demands on us in one way or another, and who make life difficult for us, because they do not allow us to express our emotions freely enough. They become our dinosaurs, but they also teach us to believe that there are other dinosaurs in our lives, because we start to feel that we cannot express our emotions freely with other people with whom we are in close contact. These people may turn out to be our difficult brother or sister, our difficult husband or wife, our difficult son or daughter, our difficult neighbours, our difficult boss at work, our difficult boss in the sky, or maybe the difficult situations we face in life. All these people and things are difficult for us, because we are brought up in ways which do not allow us to cope with them easily. We do not feel we may say what we want to.

When these dangers appear, either in reality, or merely within our thoughts, we still experience the same fight or flight response; the same chemical changes take place within our bodies and our muscles tighten up, but, so often, the chemicals do not get used up and we remain physically tense, because it is not appropriate for us to fight or run away from these people or situations. Thought can make some of us feel that we are almost constantly in danger from our own particular dinosaurs. This constant stress means that our bodies are in an almost constant state of chemical imbalance and physical tension. For much of the time we may be unaware of this, but even if we are aware of it, we may accept it as quite normal. After all, life is very stressful, we may say. Our dinosaurs come to control our lives and it is very largely the constant chemical imbalance and physical tension they cause us which eventually makes us ill.

We react to the dangers we believe we are facing in one of two ways. Either we are aggressive, which is the equivalent of fighting – we try to take control – or we are submissive, which is as near as we allow ourselves to get to running away – we hide our feelings and accept that we cannot take control. If we are submissive, we may submit and accept with good grace, or we may submit and accept with bad grace, but we accept. The less control we have over our lives, the less confidence we shall have in ourselves and the more we shall lose our sense of self-esteem. We can even come to feel that life is not really worth living.

Some of us are aggressive all the time; some of us are submissive all the time; some oscillate from one reaction to the other and there are, of course, degrees of aggressiveness and degrees of submissiveness. The words aggressive and submissive may sound derogatory. To be aggressive or submissive may not always be desirable, but these are learned reactions and I use the words in their descriptive sense. To say that someone is too submissive, in particular, can make them sound a bit of a wimp and a failure. Submissiveness can mean cringing in a corner, but this is an extreme reaction to danger. Submissiveness will often mean looking after the needs of others, to the exclusion of your own needs, perhaps coping with life and the family and with all the family's problems. It will often mean doing things for others, which, at least subconsciously, you do not really want to do. It may mean agreeing to do these things with a smile on your face and with every show of willingness. You may even believe that you really want to do these things and do them with great enthusiasm, because it feels right that you should do them. It can make you feel good to do your 'duty' in this way. If mum and dad bring you up to be nice to other people all the time, it can feel selfish and self-indulgent to look after yourself.

These lessons are often passed on from generation to generation, which is why illnesses sometimes seem to run in families. The family develops a tendency to suffer from a particular illness; some members of the family will inherit a greater tendency than others. We do not all inherit exactly the same physical and mental characteristics from our parents. If the family can be taught to face up to life in less stressful ways, the family will develop a tendency not to acquire the particular illness, rather than a tendency to have it. Science's answer is to want to try genetic engineering. If we are not careful, we shall produce a Frankenstein monster.

When we lived purely by instinct and could not think, we had only the physical stress which all animals have, if they are to survive in a more or less hostile environment. Learning to think not only allowed us to start worrying about our personal dinosaurs, it also allowed us to develop our brains and produce today's potentially very stressful modern industrial society, which can inflict considerably more physical and mental stress upon us. Our modern and very materialistic society has also helped us to lose sight of our place within nature and to lose sight of the spiritual element in our lives. Because of the ways in which we are brought up and because of the world in which we live, we may now have a great deal of almost continuous physical, mental and spiritual stress in our lives and we need to learn how to deal with this stress, if it is not going to make us ill.

The first symptoms of long term, low level stress may show up as fatigue, a tendency to get coughs and colds and viral infections too easily, general depression, headaches, back pains and limb pains, stomach and bowel disorders, respiratory disorders, allergies, skin complaints, and the like. Myalgic encephalomyelitis – ME – or post viral fatigue syndrome, as it is sometimes called, is just another example of long term, low level stress. If the stress levels are not too high and if we are not too continuously under stress, we may get away with just these symptoms. If the stress levels are too high and if the stress does continue for too long, then we may develop more serious illness, ulcers, heart disease, arthritis, multiple sclerosis, cancer, or whatever it may be.

2

What is Holistic Healing?

It is because physical, mental and spiritual stress are all present in our lives that they will all normally be present in our illness. That is why the holistic approach to illness wants to look with the patient – who is going to be actively involved throughout – at the physical, mental and spiritual stress in the patient's life. Holistic healing teaches the patient to understand physical, mental and spiritual stress and it teaches the patient how to deal with these stresses from the past, present and future. It therefore looks at the whole being, body, mind and spirit, and this is the initial 'whole' in 'holistic'. We talk about body and mind and spirit as if they were three totally separate parts of ourselves. We have to do this to describe them, but they are inextricably inter-twined in our whole being; we do not exist as three parts, each leading its own independent existence. Holistic healing teaches patients how to heal themselves, by teaching them how to handle stress, and it therefore teaches them how to prevent a recurrence of illness. It is about healing and about prevention, but it is also about a way of life. The ultimate 'whole' in 'holistic' is the wholeness of our human being within the wholeness of Creation.

Holistic healing is based on two simple facts. The first concerns the power of the mind. When our mind tells our body there is danger present, the body obeys and prepares us immediately for fight or flight. It is because we so often worry about things and unconsciously keep on

sending danger messages to our bodies that many of us
eventually become ill. We need consciously to change the
message and say to ourselves that there is no real danger,
and then the body will cease to put us into a state of
chemical imbalance and physical tension. We have truly
to believe that there is no real danger, physical, mental or
spiritual, if the message is to be effective, and initially this
may not be so easy. In the final analysis, however, it is
very often largely our mind which makes our body ill and
we can therefore consciously use this powerful mind, both
to make us well again and to keep us well. It can be
difficult for many people to believe that mental stress can
make them physically ill and that it can give them cancer.
It can therefore be equally difficult for them to believe that
they have the power to heal themselves. They do not allow
themselves to believe that they could do it, which is often
the greatest obstacle to their recovery.

The second fact on which holistic healing is based is
that our bodies know how to heal themselves and will
heal themselves if we give them relatively stress free
conditions. No surgeon would be able to perform another
operation, if our bodies did not heal themselves. We need
to have our wounds kept clean, bound up and protected
for a time – we need to give them relatively stress free
conditions – but then they heal. We accept that this will
happen and it does, even though there may be no really
good reason why it should. It is quite miraculous, when
you stop to think about it. Our bodies do have the most
fantastic self-healing powers. They know how to heal
themselves, and they will, providing we give them relatively stress free conditions.

Holistic healing seeks to harness together the immense
self-healing powers of the body with the equally immense
powers of the mind. That patients can be taught to do this
successfully, there is no doubt. If we control the stress in
our lives, we control what happens in our bodies, and we
control our health.

Holistic healing will not work, of course, if patients are

unable, or unwilling to remove the causes of the physical, mental and spiritual stress in their lives. The patient has to want to get well and has to be prepared to put in considerable time and effort into doing so. Even when the immune system is badly undermined and the patient is very ill, there can still be hope, providing the patient is prepared to put in time and effort. There are many cancer patients alive today who were originally told by their orthodox practitioners that they had only months or weeks to live, but who were helped to survive by the holistic approach. Some orthodox practitioners would claim that the patient's survival was still due purely to the orthodox treatment, the effects of which had taken rather longer than usual to show up. I doubt if any patient who had survived in this way would agree with them. Alternatively, it might be claimed that the patient was merely in remission. The patient might prefer to say that they were, at any rate for the time being, in control of their cancer.

Some patients, it is true, do seem to do fine, solely on the orthodox treatment for cancer – surgery, radiotherapy, chemotherapy, or hormone therapy – particularly if the cancer is diagnosed at a relatively early stage. There can be good reasons for this. Orthodox medicine has indeed made great strides, with better surgical and radiotherapy techniques and better mixes of chemotherapy drugs; no doubt it will improve its techniques still further. Removing a cancerous growth from the body obviously enough removes something foreign to the body, something with which the immune system is not coping. When the orthodox treatment removes this growth from the body, it therefore relieves the body of this physical stress. It may, in addition, relieve some of the patient's mental stress, because the patient knows that the orthodox treatment has removed the growth. Cancer consultants are powerful figures and they have powerful machines and drugs at their disposal. If patients have faith that they will be cured by these means, this will undoubtedly help to relieve some of the mental stress associated with their illness.

A further factor is that people who are seriously ill receive a great deal of attention, not only from doctors and nurses, but also, if they are lucky, from their family and friends. Some of us do not get enough love and attention in our lives and this can be a major cause of stress for us; illness can be a cry for love and attention. On the other hand, whilst we may in no way be seeking love and attention through our illness, the fact that we are ill may bring us more love and attention and this may also help to relieve some of our mental stress. It may be that we develop a better relationship with our husband or wife, or with other members of our family, with whom previously we had a difficult and stressful relationship. This, of course, may not only apply to patients who have purely orthodox treatment.

Similarly, many patients with life threatening illness may be brought to consider their spiritual needs, because their illness forces them to face up to the possibility of imminent death. If they gain a sense of spiritual peace, this will also help to relieve some of the stress in their lives. Again, this does not only apply to patients who have purely the orthodox treatment.

Anything which helps to relieve physical, mental or spiritual stress in the patient's life will be useful. The orthodox treatment sets out merely to deal with the physical symptoms, which are the end result of the physical, mental and spiritual stress the patient has suffered and which are the cause of the patient's illness. If, by accident or design, the orthodox treatment permanently removes sufficient stress from the patient, the patient will be cured. If it does not, the patient may go into remission for a time, but will quite possibly die sooner or later, either from a recurrence of their primary cancer, or from secondary cancer, which develops as a spread from the primary site. Unfortunately, the orthodox treatment is itself sometimes very stressful for cancer patients and, whilst it may take some stress away with one hand, it tends to give back much more with the other. Some cancer patients undoubtedly die, because the stress of their orthodox treatment is added to the stress of their illness.

Unfortunately too, the fear surrounding cancer is made much worse by the way in which some patients are rushed into orthodox treatment, as if they were likely to die if they did not get the orthodox treatment the next day. The majority of cancers will have taken years to develop to the point where they could be detected. Some will be fast growing, but many will not be, and there is no good reason for such excessive haste in these cases. Patients need to be treated as individual human beings and have their illness and possible treatment thoroughly discussed with them, so that they may fully understand all the avenues open to them before they begin treatment.

The cry for science to find a new, wonder drug cure for cancer reflects misunderstanding of the causes of cancer. The millions of pounds spent on research into cancer and other chronic illnesses reflects the belief that physical illness can always be cured purely by physical means, if only the right physical means can be found. Science likes tangible things which it can see and measure. Mental and spiritual stress do not come within this category and orthodox medicine tends to disregard them. The money spent on cancer research may well bring further improvements in current orthodox techniques and may well improve initial survival rates, which can only be welcome. If patients still continue their stressful ways after their orthodox treatment, however, they will still be candidates for a recurrence of their illness, however good the initial orthodox treatment may be.

A few patients do choose not to have the orthodox treatment, but to rely solely on the holistic approach, maybe because they understand that their illness is not just a physical thing to be dealt with in a physical way. It may seem a brave decision, though some patients will say that they are just too scared by what is on offer from the orthodox treatment. It is possible to learn to control cancer using only the holistic approach; some do it. The danger lies in the fact that the stressful habits, which will have contributed in large measure to the patient getting cancer, will be deeply ingrained habits and it will be difficult to change them and difficult to change them quickly. That it can sometimes be done, there is no doubt.

The vast majority of patients, of course, are only told about the orthodox treatment for cancer. I believe that all patients should be given the opportunity to learn holistic methods of self-healing, alongside the orthodox treatment. Preferably they should start to learn these holistic methods before they begin any orthodox treatment – and this will not take up a great deal of time. They may then stand up better to the treatment, they may recover more quickly and, as they progress, they should learn to prevent a recurrence of their illness in the future.

At the moment there is still far too much fear attached to cancer for the holistic approach to be a viable alternative to the orthodox treatment for the vast majority of cancer patients. It may be that it will never be a viable alternative for most patients. It can be a vitally important complementary approach for all patients, with the orthodox treatment buying time for the holistic lessons to be fully learned and fully put into practice. Many of those who now die, do not need to.

I hope that this book will help to dispel some of the fear attached to cancer by looking at the causes of illness and by showing how much we can all do for ourselves, not only to make ourselves better, if we are ill, but also to prevent ourselves falling ill in the first place. When the National Health Service was set up in 1948, the pious hope was voiced that society would gradually be made so healthy that the N.H.S. would virtually wither away. Regrettably, neither the N.H.S. nor the medical profession seem to have much idea of how to prevent the illness which fills the hospitals and the doctors' surgeries. The general policy has been, and continues to be, to try to pick up the pieces after the event, rather than to prevent it taking place in the first instance. Treating the end results of stress does not usually remove that stress, or its causes. Treating purely the symptoms of illness in physical ways, and neglecting the causes of that illness, often largely mental, is misguided. With this sort of policy, the N.H.S. will never have the money or resources to cope. More and more money goes on increasingly sophisticated and expensive techniques and drugs, the vast majority of which would not be necessary if we were taught to look after ourselves properly in the first place.

It is gratifying to see that interest is now being shown by some members of the orthodox medical community in at least some aspects of the holistic approach. Holistic healing does not require expensive machinery, nor does it require expensive drugs. It does require a fundamentally different approach to illness and to the patient.

So much for the scene setting. I should like to look in more detail now at the mental, physical and spiritual stress factors behind illness, starting with the mental factors, because these are so often what lie at the root of serious illness. Then I will give some examples of how the various factors influence and lead to different illnesses, and then discuss the holistic methods of dealing with each of the three sets of stress factors. It is not a complicated story.

3

The Mental Stress Factors behind Illness

We all get some degree of stress in our lives, but some of us are undoubtedly born more sensitive to it than others. It is not the amount of stress we get in our lives, but how we react to it that is important. What influences our reactions to stress more than anything else is the upbringing we receive from our parents, for it is this which teaches us how to react to life and to the society in which we live. As young babies, we probably have only two feelings, comfort and discomfort. When we are hungry, or wet or dirty, or too hot or too cold, we feel discomfort and we make this known by crying out and waving our arms and legs about. We are born with some aggression in us, so that we may survive. If we are lucky, our aggression makes mum or dad pick us up, do whatever is necessary, and make us comfortable again. As we grow and develop our ability to think, 'comfort' becomes happiness, but 'discomfort', or the possibility of 'discomfort', becomes danger. We learn to react to danger, either more or less aggressively, or more or less submissively.

In an ideal upbringing, we shall get unconditional love to start with all the time, so that we find the world a safe place to live in. Then gradually we shall be made to wait sometimes to be picked up and have our needs met, because we have to learn that other people also have needs, which may take priority over our own. We shall learn that this does not mean that we are any less loved than before. Then we shall be taught how to satisfy our own needs, in a balanced way, bearing others in mind. We shall be taught that it is just as wrong always to fulfill our needs to the exclusion of the needs of others, as it is always to fulfil others' needs to the exclusion of our own. A balanced upbringing makes for an enjoyable life.

Babies who are left to cry until they stop will learn to believe that there is little control they can have over their lives. The natural aggression they show by crying is what they need to survive. If this does not get them what they want, which is to be picked up and made comfortable, they may learn to be passive and submissive to whatever life throws at them. They may well become the sort of people who always seem to be suffering from coughs and colds and odd minor infections. Their lives will seem vaguely unsatisfactory to them for much of the time. They may make unsatisfactory marriages and help their children to do the same. They are not taught to take responsibility for their lives and make things happen that they wish to happen. They are drifters in life and they are candidates for illness. So too, of course, are children who are over-disciplined and never allowed to cry.

The amount of love we receive as babies is therefore vital. The opposite end of the scale to unconditional love is no love at all. No love means, 'you are not wanted; do not exist' – which is a very harsh command. At a much lesser level, a child may still sense some restraint on the part of its mother, if the mother has a subconscious fear of being unable to cope with the child, shut away in the house, largely on her own, as many mothers are today. The 'experts' offer conflicting advice on how to bring up a child and this further undermines her confidence. She may try to be a good mother and may appear to outsiders to be so. Music can be technically perfect, but if it is not played from the heart it will probably not reach the heart of the audience. Babies are nothing if not instinctively perceptive. At another level, there may be the realisation that the child, which the parents thought they wanted, is not really wanted after all. Many a puppy, which looked so appealing in the shop window, is found at home to be messy, noisy and time consuming. The child may perhaps be tolerated, but it is not really loved.

Unconditional love comes from the natural bonding which normally takes place between mother and child at birth. Autistic children can sometimes seem to be a case where successful bonding has not been fully achieved, or where it has broken down. It has been shown that, where the bond can be established, or re-established, between mother and child, a cure can be effected. It requires the painful experience for the mother of having to hold the child and keep forcing it to make eye contact, despite all the child's struggles, physical and vocal, to avoid this. The mother will probably need considerable support from experienced helpers, and from her husband, if he can be persuaded to be with her. It has been proved to work in some cases, when carried out for a sufficient length of time.

Autistic children are clearly not 'in touch' with their parents, or anyone else. The autistic traits of withdrawal and of periodic aggression are, however, the same flight and fight reactions we all display when we are faced with danger, or what we believe to be danger. It is also possible that dietary factors may play at least a contributory role. It is known that some children are so affected by chemical additives in food and drink that they become hyperactive. Other chemicals may affect the chemical activity of the brains of other children in other ways.

The strength of the need for bonding is clearly apparent in animals. Ducklings, for instance, will bond with a human being and treat the human as their mother, if their real mother is taken away from them at birth. They will even attempt to bond with a cardboard cutout of their mother, if that is all that is on offer. In so-called primitive societies, babies are with their mothers from birth and are even carried around on the mother's back whilst she is working. We may dump baby in a cot in another ward when baby is born, where it can cry with lots of other babies, whilst mum gets some rest. Production-line methods of childbirth may mean that mum gets more rest. They are of doubtful benefit to baby.

If we receive too little love in our childhood, it is bound to affect us and it will have effects on our health at some time during our lives. The less love we receive as young children, the greater the mental stress we suffer. It will also affect the way we relate to others later in life. We may find it difficult to give love, or we may try to compensate by giving too much love. It will be difficult for us to get the balance right – which will be stressful both for us and for the others concerned.

The first weeks of our lives merge into the first years, and the learning process continues for us as we adapt to what our parents seem to want from us. We depend on them for all our needs – in a word, for survival – and we seek their love and therefore do what seems necessary to us to obtain that love; that is the price we have to pay to 'buy' this love. We can get all sorts of messages from our parents, telling us what they want, and these messages will depend on what sort of messages they got from their parents during their childhood, and on any lessons they may have learned in later life. All these messages will dictate how safe or how dangerous we shall find our lives to be, and how much enjoyment or otherwise we shall have in our lives.

The messages may tell us,

> 'get them before they get you', or 'keep still and they
> may not notice you';
> 'be a winner', or 'be a loser';
> 'hurry up', or 'let's take the scenic route';
> 'grow up and be independent', or 'be mummy's little
> boy/daddy's little girl';
> 'be bold and sexy', or 'be sweet and demure';
> 'be a saint', or 'be a sinner';
> 'look after number one', or 'look after everyone else';
> 'look after me', or 'get out of my way';

'everything in its place and a place for everything',
   or 'let it all hang out';
'least said soonest mended', or 'get it off your chest';
'it is your duty to', or 'let's play truant today';
'life's a ball', or 'life is hell';
'enjoy yourself', or 'have a miserable time'.

Messages may sometimes be given to us directly, but will
more often be given to us indirectly; we often learn by
example. If they are repeated often enough, we shall get
the message. Sometimes we may get one set of messages
from mum and a different set from dad. This makes life
more confusing and gives us a lot more stress. Sometimes,
when we are a bit older and feel capable of taking our own
decisions, we may decide that we do not really like what
we have been told to do, and we may go off and do just the
opposite. Some of us stay as rebels all our lives. Some
rebel for a time and then fall back into line.

What the messages teach us is how much, or how little,
we are allowed to express our natural emotions, initially
with our parents, but later on also with the other people in
our lives. An uninhibited child expresses its emotions
quite freely, through the use of both sound and physical
movement, and, having got rid of its emotions, it gets on
with its life. If we are uninhibited, we can roar and shake
with anger, and we can roar and shake with laughter; we
can moan and shake with fear, and we can moan and
shake with sorrow. Some volatile families are like this and
express their emotions very readily and in very voluble
fashion. They do not suppress and hang on to their
emotions. Most of us are brought up to be rather more
restrained and a bit more submissive, because that is
what mum and dad want. We are taught to suppress our
emotions at times, and a certain amount of discipline is no
bad thing. The dangers come when we are taught by mum
and dad to suppress our emotions too much and be too
submissive, for this can become very stressful for us.

In some families it can be almost a sin to express anger at any time. It may be a very religious family, but not necessarily so. It is just not done to express anger in any shape or form. Anger is viewed as a negative, nasty and base emotion, which must always be suppressed. In some families, the emphasis is on sweetness and light, with love flowing in all directions; anger just does not exist. Some of the children in these families accept the saintly role in life. Others may find this perfectionist medicine rather too sickly and rebel instead, taking up what seem to them to be more interesting pursuits, such as drugs, drink, sex and crime. If the messages we send to any of our children are having the wrong effect, maybe we should consider modifying the messages. Perfectionist messages often create difficulties; we all need to let our hair down from time to time. Even Jesus was prepared to turn the water into wine, so that the wedding guests could go on enjoying themselves.

In some other families it is not done to express fear; with others it is sorrow. Fear and sorrow are considered to be inferior feelings, only shown by lesser mortals and everyone has to put on a brave face, put these feelings behind them, and carry on as if nothing had happened. There are even families where there is little time for laughter. It may be the puritan ethic, which thinks that we are not on this earth to enjoy ourselves. It may be that life seems very scary and dangerous and that there is no room for laughter.

These families try to teach their children to suppress their emotions and be submissive in the face of the dangers from the difficult people and situations they come across in life – and they often succeed. The submissiveness indeed confirms that these people and situations are difficult. If those concerned could express themselves freely, without inhibition, there would be no difficulties. Other children are taught to be aggressive as a way of dealing with these dangers. Again, the aggression itself confirms that these people and situations are difficult. Our own aggression can be justified, if we feel that others are being aggressive towards us.

Both submissiveness and aggressiveness are ways of covering up the fear of the difficulties and dangers. If they are too many and too persistent, consciously or unconsciously, we shall also feel anger at the ways in which we are treated by life and by those around us; consciously or unconsciously, we shall also feel sorrow that we do not get more fun out of life. Others are more in control of our lives than we are. Whether we are submissive or aggressive, the message we send to our body is that there is danger. The body reacts with a flow of adrenalin and with physical tension. If we do this year in and year out, we shall eventually become ill.

Serious illness is a little bit like serious earthquakes; both are to do with the build-up of huge pressures. Earthquakes occur when two sections of land on either side of a geological fault need to move in relationship to each other. They can do this in frequent, small moves, which may sometimes cause minor upsets and may sometimes be almost imperceptible. On the other hand, they may become locked together for a long period of time, so that huge pressures build up, which can only be released through a major earthquake. We may express and let go our emotions, all the time, as we need to, and this may occasionally cause us minor upsets with other people and will sometimes pass almost unnoticed by others. Alternatively, we can suppress our emotions for a long period of time, so that huge pressures build up, which lead eventually to the onset of major physical illness. Real earthquakes cause damage when the pressures are released, of course. We cause damage to ourselves, when we do not release our emotional pressures.

Mental stress is not the only factor in cancer, or in other serious illness, but it will be a very major factor in the vast majority of cases of serious illness, including cancer. If we send danger messages to our bodies, they react appropriately. We have to learn consciously to change the messages and, to do that, we have to learn consciously to change the ways in which we think, speak and act.

4

The Physical Stress Factors behind Illness

The first physical stress factor which affects us is the family background from which we come. We cannot choose our parents, nor can we choose the family into which we are born. If our family is an unhealthy one, we start off with this bad luck factor. There may be nothing we can do about the family history of bad health before we are born. There is an immense amount we can do, as we grow up, to see that we do not suffer the same unhealthy fate and to see that any children we produce do not suffer the same unhealthy fate. We should all do our children a great favour if we would ensure that we are as healthy as possible, before we even contemplate having a family.

That said, not all the children in a family will necessarily inherit the same physical and mental characteristics from their parents. Even identical twins can have different temperaments and so have different health patterns in life. This happened in my own family. In this sense, what we inherit is the luck of the draw. As I said earlier, all the members of a family may inherit a tendency towards a certain illness, but some members of the family may inherit this more strongly than others. All the members of the family need to pay attention to the possibility of contracting the illness, but some need to pay extra attention to this possibility.

Thereafter, the greatest physical stress factors for us today have come about because of the industrial revolution and the more recent chemical revolution. For thousands of years mankind lived in a clean, unpolluted atmosphere. For thousands of years mankind was able to eat natural, unpolluted foods and to drink fresh water. In the very short space of the last 100–200 years, we have forced ourselves to try to adapt to very different conditions. We live and work today in a very polluted world. We know that many of the chemicals we use are toxic and that some are carcinogenic. Disposal of chemical and nuclear wastes is an increasing problem. Many now understand that decisive action is now necessary, if we are not, one day, to make the planet uninhabitable and so destroy mankind. The industrial revolution, and particularly the chemical revolution of the past 50–100 years, have much to answer for. They seemed to promise so much; there is a high price to pay. If we treat the land, the sea and the air as dustbins we shall have to pay that price.

The same chemical revolution has transformed our diet. In the beginning, man was designed to be a vegetarian. We have the long digestive tract of herbivorous animals. Meat eating animals have a short digestive tract, because meat putrefies quickly and needs to pass through it quickly. At some point, we started to kill and eat animals, maybe because herbivores have to spend a long time feeding and we decided we wanted to spend time on other things. Maybe some climatic change made our normal food short for a time and we just got used to eating meat and never went back to being herbivores. The meat, and the fruits, roots and berries we ate were at least natural products of nature. The chemical revolution changed all that. Today, seed is dressed with chemicals, ground is fertilised with them, crops are sprayed with them, harvested crops are preserved with them. Some of the chemicals leach into water supplies, to add to those from factory effluents, and the water we drink becomes polluted. Animals may be given hormones and antibiotics to make them grow more quickly and to a greater size, to produce higher yields, and to keep them 'healthy'. Traces of these chemicals can remain in the meat and milk we consume. Persistent use of antibiotics can produce stronger viruses with resistance to the antibiotics. Many animals are also reared in factory farms under very stressful conditions and inevitably some become diseased.

On top of all this, chemicals are widely used in the production of foods which go into our grocery stores and our methods of food handling are not always perfect. Much of our food is packaged, tinned, frozen or preserved in some way; it is far from being the natural food which mother nature used to provide for us. Living in towns and cities as we do, it is inevitable that our food will not always be as fresh as might be desirable. The vitamin and mineral content of many foods on offer to the public today, however, must be extremely low, if not non-existent. Some of it truly is junk food. The more polluted our food, the more likely we are to develop food allergies and intolerance to some foods – the possible fore-runners to more serious illness later on.

We are of course assured that all these chemicals are quite safe for us in the minute quantities in which they are being used in individual foods. That may be so, or it may not. It seems highly unlikely, however, that small quantities of hundreds of individually 'safe' chemicals, ingested through food, drink and the atmosphere, over a period of years, are going to be quite as safe. Occasionally it is decided that one of these 'safe' chemicals is not quite so safe after all and it is withdrawn from use. It is usually replaced by another 'safer' chemical, once again without any regard to the cocktail of chemicals we are already ingesting from other sources. The practice of irradiating food to make it safe to consume, because it may have listeria or salmonella, is an indictment of our methods of animal rearing, food production and food handling and processing. The answer is not to irradiate food, which is merely to add one more very doubtful ingredient to the cocktail, it is to clean up our methods of food production, so that the foods are safe in the first place.

We sometimes add to our physical stress by taking excessive amounts of alcohol, by smoking and by drug taking. Over-prescription of medical drugs, such as tranquillisers, can also be very harmful, and this is now more widely recognised. Unfortunately, patients can end up suffering more from the side effects of the drugs they are taking than from the original illness for which the drugs were prescribed. It is now also recognised that the long term use of hormones, both in H.R.T. – hormone replacement therapy – and the contraceptive pill, carries risks of cancer in some cases. All drugs will tend to have side effects, some more serious than others, and the long term use of drugs for any illness or condition is potentially dangerous.

Another physical stress factor for many of us is the sedentary life we lead these days. In our earliest times, we led a very active outdoor existence. There may have been dangers in our lives, but flab was not one of them. Many of us no longer take the physical care of our bodies which we need to. Our car engines often get more loving care than our bodies, which also deserve a little planned maintenance.

It all sounds a sorry tale. Luckily for us, the human body does seem to be able to adapt to some degree; we should all be dead otherwise. We are pushing our luck very hard, however. Far too many of us fall ill, with cancer, or with some other illness. If we are interested in our health, we need not only to pay attention to the mental stress factors in our lives, we must also pay attention to the physical stress factors. We need to keep a supple, fit body; we need to cleanse it and feed it as natural a diet as possible; and we need to keep the chemical pollution in our living and working environments to the lowest levels we can.

5

The Spiritual Stress Factors
behind Illness

Once we learned to think, we were able to start wondering what life was all about. There were many powerful things in nature which we could neither understand nor control. The idea of powerful gods and goddesses who could control these things must have come easily to our minds, which helped us perhaps to a sense of our place within a greater pattern of life. We also lived close to nature and must have been more aware of the passing of the seasons and of the rhythm of our lives and the world in which we lived. There was a spiritual element in our lives, however pagan that element might appear to us today. We will have accepted that this was an integral and essential part of our lives.

Today, with our modern industrial society, we seem to believe that we can control nature and the world to suit what we perceive to be our needs. What we want is paramount and we think we can ride roughshod over nature. In earliest times, we took what we needed from what she provided at the place where we were and, if we used up the supplies there, we moved on, and the place where we had been had time to recover. Progress today dictates that we often take so much from the earth, that there is no possible hope of it recovering. We believe that our knowledge and ingenuity will enable us to go on indefinitely, creating our own future and our own destiny. We may be right and we may be wrong. There is little place for God in such a scenario, it may sometimes

seem. Our continual desire for bigger and better and for
shinier and glossier takes us further and further away
from nature and from natural ways of life, and further and
further away from the idea of a Creator, who created a
totally integrated and interdependent Universe – a balanced eco system, in terms of our own planet. We have
already destroyed parts of this Universal jigsaw on our
planet and parts of the picture will never be replaced. Very
little seems sacred to us any longer, when everything
should be sacred, if we say that God created the Universe
and everything within it.

We need a spiritual element in our lives if our lives are
to have any real purpose. Life has no real purpose otherwise. Sadly, it sometimes seems to take a catastrophe for
us to realise this. A major disaster takes place and we wish
to lay flowers at the site; we pray for those who died and
for those who were bereaved; we hold memorial services
in church. For a time we are aware of our spiritual nature
and we are the better for it.

Mankind is suffering from a great lack of spirituality
and from a great excess of pride in his own abilities.
Unless we regain a goodly sense of humility, a real sense
of the ways in which everything in the world is interdependent, and a true sense of spirituality, the future of the
world must be in doubt.

We may be largely unaware of how stressful is the lack
of a spiritual dimension to our lives. The stress is there
and it will be a factor in our illness. Our illness, particularly if it is a life-threatening illness such as cancer, can
increase our spiritual stress. It can make us think that God
is not looking after us, or that God has deserted us, or
maybe even that there can be no God. If our illness brings
us to an understanding of our spiritual need, we may seek
to do something about it. Our spiritual stress may be
relieved if we come to a sense that God is still with us,
however ill we are. Our healing will be helped to that
degree.

As children, we start life with a natural sense of wonder

at everything around us in nature; we have a natural sense of spirituality. The materialistic world into which we are born soon knocks that out of us. If our horizons are limited to this materialistic world, it is very difficult for us to have any sense of 'the peace which passeth all understanding'.

6

How Stress is Involved in Illness

Before looking at how stress is involved in cancer, it is interesting to look first at how stress is involved in some other illnesses. It is even involved in the common cold. We probably all have cold germs in our bodies most of the time, but they are kept under control by our immune systems. When we are a bit under stress, physically, mentally or spiritually, the stress undermines the immune system and we then 'catch' a cold. Even if a totally new and virulent flu virus is brought into the country, not everyone who comes into contact with it will get flu – not everyone got the black plague when that was around either. This has little to do with luck. It has to do with the strength or weakness of our immune systems and the degree to which they have built up antibodies, or can quickly produce them.

It is the same for Aids patients. The more physical, mental or spiritual stress in the life of those who have acquired the Aids virus, the more likely and the more quickly they will be to develop full blown Aids. They will 'catch' the disease when the amount of stress in their lives, physical, mental, and/or spiritual, undermines their immune systems sufficiently to allow this to happen. To prevent Aids developing, it is necessary to get stress out of patients' lives and to keep it out of their lives, so that their immune systems are as strong as possible. Probably the greatest stress factor for many H.I.V. positive patients will be the knowledge that they have the Aids virus and the fear and belief that they will therefore develop full blown Aids.

It is mental stress which is so often a major factor in serious illness. With a little investigation, physical stress factors may become readily apparent, and these need to be eliminated, as do spiritual stress factors. Mental stress factors can be less immediately apparent, but can have equally, and sometimes much more harmful physical effects upon the body. I have said that mental stress revolves around the ways in which we react to the dangers we perceive in our lives; we may react more aggressively, or we may react more submissively.

Ulcer patients tend towards the submissive reaction. They therefore find it difficult to get truly angry and they worry instead about the dangers and difficulties of staying in control of their lives. The businessman who gets an ulcer probably feels that he has got a stressful job. He will almost certainly give the impression of finding it stressful and is probably not averse to letting others know what a stressful job it is. He will have been brought up by mum and dad to be a bit of a worrier. He was quite probably also brought up to be a bit of a perfectionist, which makes you worry about getting things right. Dad was probably a perfectionist as well. Perfectionists like everything neat and tidy and they can be a bit too meticulous for their own good. If you always worry about the difficulties and dangers of controlling things in your life, you may well end up with an ulcer.

Middle management is an easy place to pick up ulcers. You have to worry about looking after the staff under you, and about what senior management over you require from you. You can get kicks from both sides; both seem like dangerous dinosaurs. Worrying will of course upset your digestion, which will help you to develop an ulcer. A poor diet may speed up the process. If you take to smoking to calm your nerves, this will not help your breathing and, since you probably find it hard to breathe emotionally, sinus troubles may add to your miseries.

The aggressive reaction can show up in those with heart disease, though not everyone who is aggressive gets a heart attack, nor is everyone who gets a heart attack aggressive. As with ulcer patients, of course, smoking is not helpful; nor is eating a high cholesterol diet. These are physical factors which need to be eliminated. Those with heart disease, however, can well be those who react aggressively to their dangers. They drive themselves on relentlessly, angrily spurred on by a feeling that time is always short. Their aggressiveness will have been learned from their parents. Driving yourself on relentlessly is like running the whole time; having to win every race is bound to put a strain on your heart. A gentle jog round the highways and byways of life might be just as enjoyable and far less taxing.

An illness where both aggression and submission can play a role together is arthritis. Arthritis is an illness which afflicts many and, once again, as with all illnesses, physical factors can be involved. Excessive wear and tear of the joints is an obvious one; old age tells many of us that our joints are wearing out a bit. In Britain, the rather damp climate is another unhelpful factor. Many arthritics would fare much better in a warmer and drier climate; they can find that their arthritis gets much better when they are on their summer holiday in the Mediterranean. Some also do better after changing to a simpler and more natural whole food diet – this does not only apply to arthritics. Arthritics can suffer from constipation and a more natural diet can improve this. Some arthritics also do better taking one of the herbal or homoeopathic remedies from their health food shop. One of the best remedies often seems to be the good old fashioned cod liver oil, which many of us were given as children, though it may take some time to show results; it needs also to be combined with improved diet and other measures.

The mental stress in arthritis comes from the frustration which many arthritics seem to experience in their lives. There is some arthritis in my family. My father was

brought up by a fairly strict Victorian mother. Luckily his
father had a quiet sense of humour and a twinkle in his
eye, but it must have been a somewhat inhibiting atmosphere in which to be brought up. My mother, on the
other hand, was brought up to have rather more nervous
energy. My mother once told me, after my father had died,
that he often used to have dreams about flying and that he
had not been able to understand why. I imagine that
anyone who had been brought up by a strict Victorian
mother and had then had to go to the same office in the
West End, day in and day out for forty years, as my father
had to, would want to fly. Those in the family who inherit
too much nervous energy, which makes them want to fly,
but who also inherit too much Victorian inhibition, which
prevents them flying, are those who get arthritis.

The frustration of the arthritic can show up in the
everyday minor events of life; the milkman who inevitably calls just after you have gone upstairs to make the
beds; the kids who always leave their rooms in a mess; the
way the toast always falls on the floor butter side down.
These things are indeed annoying, but the arthritic can
find them just that extra bit frustrating. Arthritics may be
able to express their anger and frustration, but they often
cannot let it go and it lingers on in their minds and
continues to frustrate them. We can get situations in our
lives that we would like to get away from, maybe a job
which we find frustrating, or a personal relationship,
perhaps a marriage which we find frustrating, or maybe
our relationship with our parents stifles us in some way.
We are locked into the situation, however, perhaps by
financial considerations, by the mortgage, by the pension,
by the children, by fear of what leaving the situation
might bring upon us, or perhaps just because we feel
unable to deal with the difficult person or persons concerned.

We get arthritis in the moving parts of the body, the
hands, which would like to strangle the milkman, or the
kids, or the toast, or life, but can't; the legs that would like

to move away from frustrating situations, but can't. Aggression may make us express anger and send tension into our bodies, but inhibition, which is a form of submission, prevents us taking the necessary action and letting go the anger and tension. We try to control our lives through aggression, but find that we must submit and accept many things which we do not wish to. It is no wonder we find it frustrating.

Arthritics, like ulcer patients, can also be perfectionists. It is because arthritics express their anger in one way or another, but are frustrated when they cannot control things, in preference to worrying and suppressing their anger, that they get arthritis rather than ulcers.

Multiple sclerosis patients also suffer from frustration in their lives, though they tend to the more submissive approach to their difficulties. They often seem to have a compulsive need to push themselves too hard on occasion, though they usually know that this will make them feel worse afterwards. This is sometimes rationalised as a need to cram as much into life as possible, before the disease becomes too crippling. M.S. patients are told that they will almost certainly get worse through the years and they come to believe this, which makes it difficult for them to believe that they can ever get any better. The periodic show of compulsiveness may be baffling to those close to the patient. It can appear to be a subconscious cry for love and attention. Maybe M.S. patients did not get as much love as they needed from one or other parent during their childhood. Maybe, as grownups, they now feel they are not getting as much love as they need, either within their marriages, or within their lives generally. Maybe they perceive that they are getting love now, but it still somehow does not compensate them enough for the love they lost in their childhood. Periodically, their need for more love wells up and they start to drive themselves on in an apparent attempt to prove that they are worthy to receive childhood love. Since we cannot have our childhood over again, they are bound to fail in their endeavours. Every time they do so, the stress seems literally to get on their nerves, by eating away, like an intermittent form of cancer, at the myelin sheath surrounding their nerves. They also get blood seepages at the points of damage. We speak of our heart bleeding in sympathy for someone. M.S. patients seem to bleed in sympathy for themselves and for their inability to achieve the childhood love they crave.

It would be very nice if we all got all the love we needed, both as children and as grownups. Unfortunately, others, including members of our own families, do not always love us perfectly. We, however, do not always love others perfectly ourselves. They are not saints, and neither are we, and we do not have to try to be. M.S. patients cannot get what subconsciously they appear periodically to want, but, whilst this stresses and frustrates them, because, like arthritis patients, they have to put up with it, they appear to suppress their anger and in some cases not even acknowledge that they feel anger. As with other illnesses, dietary and other physical factors can play some part and physical factors need to be taken into consideration.

M.S. might be termed an intermittent illness, which flares up whenever the patients feel a compulsive need to stress themselves for a time. Cancer, in contrast, is an illness which, in most cases, appears to come from the much more constant stress to which the patients submit themselves and feel they must accept. As with all other illnesses, physical factors can be a contributory element and these need to be eliminated where necessary. There are various things which we know to be carcinogenic. Excessive smoking is one example. If I am born with a strong constitution, do not have any great mental or spiritual stress in my life, smoke fifty cigarettes a day, but smoke purely because I enjoy smoking, the physical stress of smoking fifty cigarettes a day may be enough to give me emphysema, but not enough to give me cancer. If I have the same strong constitution, but have a bit too much mental and spiritual stress in my life, and still smoke fifty cigarettes a day, the physical stress of smoking fifty cigarettes a day, plus the mental and spiritual stress in my life, may be enough to give me cancer. If I smoke five hundred cigarettes a day, it probably will not matter how strong my constitution is, nor how much mental and spiritual stress I have in my life, I shall inevitably get cancer. The physical stress of smoking five hundred cigarettes a day is going to be too much stress for anybody's immune system. Very few people smoke five hundred cigarettes a day and very few people get cancer, or any other serious illness, purely from physical causes.

The same argument applies equally to too much asbestos dust, too much radiation, too much of certain chemicals which are carcinogenic, or too much of anything, or any combination of things, which are carcinogenic. Above certain levels, they will almost certainly cause cancer. Below those levels, they may be a contributory factor in the cancer, depending on the constitution of the person concerned and on how much additional stress that person has in their life. All things carcinogenic, or potentially carcinogenic, are best avoided completely, if possible. The risk of cancer for those on hormone replacement therapy, or the contraceptive pill, will be increased proportionately by the amount of mental and spiritual stress they have in their lives. Any other physical factor, such as smoking, will also increase the risk.

The mental factors in cancer, as with other illnesses, are to do with the difficult people and situations we find in our lives and the ways in which we have been brought up to deal with these dangers. Cancer patients normally react to them too submissively by accepting and putting up with them, because this is what their parents teach them to do. Real aggression and anger are not allowed, so the only alternative is to go on continually accepting whatever happens. Some accept with good grace and appear to their friends to be coping well with life. Others accept far less willingly, but, although they find their lives unhappy as a result, they still go on doing what they were told to do.

The stress for cancer patients is a much more constant stress, however little they may sometimes be aware of it.

One patient of mine, who was a businessman, found his retirement a difficult situation to handle. He had evidently been taught to go out into the world and succeed. He did and had a successful business career, though he told me that he found his work stressful; he had not been taught to be aggressively successful and have no qualms about it. When he retired, however, he found that he had nothing to do, because, unfortunately, he had not been taught by his parents that he was occasionally allowed to take time off for play. His work had become his whole life and when he stopped work, he ceased to have any particular reason for being around; he ceased, in his own eyes, to have any importance. He lost his self-esteem and he lost his sense of purpose in life. Within a couple of years he developed brain cancer. Perhaps, symbolically, he no longer needed his brain.

This businessman seemed to most of his friends to be an active, outgoing sort of person and it might be easy to make the mistake of thinking that here was a man who was not suppressing his emotions. The person who is taught to go out into the world and succeed will almost inevitably be taught not to show fear or weakness. A bold face can cover up fear and tears – for little boys don't cry, if they want to appear to be big boys – and we all know that big boys don't cry. In the end, this businessman, who was not really aggressive, could not summon up enough anger and aggression to do something about his difficult situation and just accepted and gave in to it.

The difficult people in our lives are very often members of our own family. One lady patient had looked after her mother for many years and, when her mother died, was left the bulk of the mother's estate. She was immediately accused by her sister of having influenced the mother into leaving her so much. She was deeply distressed by this accusation, which she felt was entirely without foundation, but she was unable to face up to the situation and

unable to face her sister. She developed cancer of the eye –
which maybe helped her not to see this painful situation.

Another lady found difficulties with her children. She
had been brought up, as many ladies are, to believe that
she had to spend most of her time looking after other
people, and she did this with great enthusiasm and
seemed to enjoy doing her duty in this way. All her
friends thought she coped with life very well and were
always roping her in to help. Unfortunately, she also spent
a lot of time looking after her own children and she was
aware that this did upset her, because she felt that they
were now quite old enough to look after themselves and
leave her more time to have fun on her own. Her children
were by this time grown up with children of their own,
but they still expected mum to be at their beck and call,
and she did not feel able to tell them to leave her in peace.
Eventually she developed breast cancer. The breast has
nurturing connotations and this lady certainly found it
difficult to nurture herself.

Husbands can also be difficult. One lady who also
developed breast cancer, was so afraid of her husband that
she told me she did not want him to know that she was
coming for counselling and healing. She clearly found it
difficult to get her own needs fulfilled. The breast also has
sexual connotations, as do some other organs of the body,
and it is going to be difficult to have a satisfactory sexual
relationship with such a difficult spouse.

Wives too can be difficult, though in the case I am
thinking of, it was not only the husband who found his
wife difficult, the children of the marriage also found her
difficult. When mum got going, everyone ducked for
cover. This gentleman developed stomach cancer; he
agreed that he had a lot in life that he could not stomach.

One lady patient told me that she had difficulties with
both her parents. Her father was a strict disciplinarian,
which aroused fear and anger in her. Her mother, who
was also in fear of the husband, expected her daughter to
look after her and fuss over her, in compensation for the

love she did not receive in sufficient quantity from her husband. The patient developed cancer of the pancreas.

The parents of another patient parted shortly after she was born and later divorced. She never knew her father and this upset and saddened her, because she felt that he did not wish to acknowledge her. She did not get on with the man her mother subsequently married and felt that her mother gave more attention to the new husband than to her. She later married herself, but she lacked confidence in herself and even felt that she was not very attractive, which was not true. A few years into her marriage she developed leukaemia.

Then there was the gentleman who, in a sense, found everybody in life difficult. He was brought up in a very inhibited, self-contained family, and he told me that they had had very few, if any, friends. Naturally enough, the gentleman in question also found it hard to make friends and, over the years, this became more and more stressful for him. Occasionally he would lose his temper about something or other and fly off the handle, but immediately he would feel guilty and submissively bottle up his anger again. He developed cancer of the bowel. Life for him was a pain in the butt.

It was also for another lady, who had various stressful family situations throughout her life. She told me that what really angered her, looking back over the years, was that she had always had to do 'the sensible thing'; she never felt that she had really enjoyed herself in life. In fact this lady did not have cancer of the bowel, she had ovarian cancer.

Another gentleman who did have bowel cancer was a musician in a symphony orchestra. The stress for him was feeling that he had to produce the perfect performance every time. You are only as good as your last performance, he told me. It gave him an almost impossible standard to meet. Life for him was certainly a pain in the butt.

To many it may seem too simplistic to imply a link between cancer of the bowel and life being a pain in the butt, or to say that a patient has cancer of the stomach because he has things in his life he cannot stomach. In some ways it obviously is. The person with bowel cancer who does find life a pain in the butt also has a lot in life they cannot stomach, yet they do not have stomach cancer; they may not be able to breathe emotionally, yet they do not have lung cancer; they may not be able to express themselves as they would wish, yet they do not have cancer of the throat or mouth; they may have things in their life they cannot look at, yet they do not have cancer of the eye. In this sense the analogies are simplistic. It is often very helpful, on the other hand, for patients to consider their cancer in these ways, because if they apply, this can help them to understand why they have cancer.

In many cases of course, where for instance patients have leukaemia, or lymphoma, or melanoma, or cancer in some other organs and parts of the body, there is no obvious analogy to be drawn, though life, or some aspects of life, will be a pain in the butt to all these patients. It may just be that the cancer merely appears first in a weak spot in the patient's body. Orthodox medicine needs to know exactly where the cancerous cells are located, because it wishes to treat these symptoms of the illness. It is of less importance to holistic healing to know with pinpoint accuracy where the patient has cancer cells, interesting and useful though this may be as a topic for discussion. The basic cause of the cancer does not lie in the bowel, or stomach, or wherever the patient has cancer. Holistic healing treats the whole person who happens to have a very serious illness called cancer and who happens to have it in a certain area of the body. It is the whole person that is sick and it is the whole person that needs treating. Holistic and other healers should, of course, always insist on knowing the diagnosis given to their patients by their doctors and should not attempt to diagnose themselves. Doctors are today's authorised diagnosticians; healers are not.

All the cancer patients I have mentioned did have

stressful lives, but what made their lives really stressful, and what they all had in common, was the degree to which they accepted too submissively that they had to put up with this stress and could do little or nothing to protest about it. Again, I emphasise that I do not use the word submissive in any derogatory sense. Virtually all of us learn, early on, that we have to put up with some things in life and accept some things we would prefer not to have to accept, if we are to get the love we need, initially from our parents, and later from others. It is the degree to which we feel forced to 'buy' love in this way which is important. Cancer patients are taught by their parents that it is their duty to accept without protest whatever life throws at them and this is what they do, whether they appear to do this gladly, or with less good will. None of them seems able really to protest at the way in which they are not allowed to have control over their lives and must go on doing their prescribed duty, either largely suppressing the anger they wish to express, or making believe that they have no anger to express. Where cancer patients usually differ from other patients with other illnesses is that they suppress their anger to the point where, consciously or subconsciously, they lose their sense of self-esteem, because, at some level, they know that they are not in control of their lives. They also lose, or start to lose, their sense that life has a worthwhile purpose for them, because, if you have so little control over your life, it can cease to have much purpose for you. Some patients lose so much self-esteem that they will even say that they do not like themselves. It is an indication of how little control they feel they have over their destinies.

Although cancer patients may lose a sense of purpose in life, they are not suicidal. Suicide, or attempted suicide, is an aggressive act against the self and cancer patients are more submissive than aggressive. Cancer patients submit to their difficulties, because that is what their parents taught them to do and, having been brought up to do this, they go on doing it for as long as they can.

Sometimes a recent traumatic event in the cancer patient's life can seem to be linked to the onset of their illness. This event will be a loss of some kind, a bereavement, a divorce, the last child leaving home, redundancy, retirement, or something similar. In the case of a fast growing cancer, the event may be some six months before cancer was diagnosed. With slower growing cancers, it can be eighteen months to two years before. This event may be interesting in itself, but, in fact, it is merely the last stressful straw which breaks the camel's back; the final thing which convinces the patient – again perhaps subconsciously – that life is not worth living. Patients have to be taught how to remove the large pile of straw which they have been piling onto their backs over a long period of time, and they have to be taught how to stop piling new straw onto their backs.

With some patients there is no apparent 'one major event' which triggers off their cancer. The straw piles up slowly on their backs and gradually the patient comes to say, as one minor thing after another goes wrong for them, 'it's the story of my life'. Cancer patients can sometimes feel like the person who was told, 'smile, things might be worse'; so they smiled and things got worse. Since cancer patients have been brought up to accept their mishaps, this is the sort of person they are, and they can feel that they must be true to themselves. They may not at first feel that they can change, even when this is suggested to them.

What illness can do – and what it will continue to do, if we let it – is to protect us and save us from having to face up to our difficulties, and from having to deal with and get rid of them. We may protect ourselves psychologically, and seem to gain certain advantages this way, but, in so doing, we harm ourselves physically. Just occasionally illness does serve directly as a means of obtaining love and attention, which the patient does not normally get in life. The patient prefers to remain ill so as to keep this love and attention. 'Can't heal myself' can sometimes mean 'won't heal myself'.

The sad truth is that, most often, it is we ourselves who make ourselves ill, which may seem a foolish thing to do. We do it, because as grown ups we continue the habit we were taught in childhood of not releasing and getting rid of our natural emotions. Our illness is a measure of how well we were taught to do this and how well we absorbed the lesson. If our parents were aware of what, inadvertently, they were doing to us, and if we were aware of what, inadvertently, we were doing to ourselves, perhaps we might all alter our ways. As grown ups, we at least are free to change the habit we learned in childhood – if we wish to.

7

Getting the Pile of Straw off your Back

Many cancer patients express enormous relief when they find a counsellor who will truly listen to them, let them unburden their soul, and understand what they feel. Orthodox medical practice often does not give them the opportunity to do this. You may have experienced this yourself. The traditional counselling skills of listening and responding appropriately are a necessary first therapy for cancer patients. This alone is not enough however. Cancer patients then also need prompt, direct and proper instruction in how to deal with the stress in their lives. Here, inevitably, the teacher has to rely to some extent on the patient; patients cannot be forced to come along for counselling. The amount of counselling you need is something which should be discussed between you and your counsellor. A good counsellor will understand your particular needs. A good counsellor will also understand how and when to vary the emphasis of approach to you, the patient.

It is not difficult to discover where the difficulties lie in anyone's life. A short discussion with them will quickly show where the difficulties lie. What were, or are, the relationships like with father and mother, brothers and sisters, husband or wife, sons and daughters? This will reveal how any of us were taught to face up to life and why we were not allowed to express our emotions freely enough, if this is the case. It will reveal why we are the person we are and why maybe we feel that we must continue to be the person we are. It should not be difficult to get you to understand why you have cancer.

Having established with you just where you are at the moment, it is then a question of getting you to move forward from this position. If you have followed certain behavioural paths in life, which have been too stressful and have therefore made you ill, it is easy enough for you to understand that it might be no bad thing to consider changing direction. To talk of change is very easy. To effect change in these circumstances can be more difficult. You have to learn how to change the deeply ingrained habits of perhaps half a life time. Mum and dad brought us up to obey certain rules – to suppress certain emotions. Mum and dad may be long dead, but their voices still reach us; we are inevitably largely the persons they brought us up to be. It is they who taught us to act aggressively, or submissively to what they taught us to view as the difficult and dangerous people and situations in our lives. Effectively, they created our dinosaurs for us and they taught us how to react to them. They may themselves, of course, be the main dinosaurs in our lives, the people against whom we do, or should, feel most anger. It is important to recognise and acknowledge who or what are the dinosaurs in your life and to recognise and acknowledge that you are entitled to feel anger against them, if they have made your life unnecessarily unhappy in the past, or if they are making your life unnecessarily unhappy now. Many patients do not seem to realise just how much stress they have been under during their lives.

To get you to move forward from your present position, two things are necessary. Firstly, you have to learn to get rid of the past accumulation of emotions you have suppressed over the years, a great deal of which will be anger, because this is what has stressed you and made you ill – this is the pile of straw which broke the camel's back. Secondly, you have to learn to gain control over your life, so that you do not need to suppress your emotions and stress yourself in the future – you have to learn how to stop piling straw onto your back. Let us look at the first step, getting the pile of straw off your back.

Some patients find it difficult to acknowledge anger in themselves. 'I'm just not an angry sort of person', they say, which, of course, nicely confirms how well they have absorbed the lesson they were taught in childhood that anger should never be expressed. Anger is natural to us. We aggressively display our displeasure as babies, as soon as we suffer discomfort, so as to let mum know that something is amiss. We need some aggression in life, if we are to survive. Anger can only be expressed, or suppressed; it cannot be wiped off the map of human existence. If you suppress your anger, it merely becomes subconscious anger and it is no good trying to convince yourself that you are a truly laid back, relaxed human being, if subconsciously you are full of anger. You may be able to fool your conscious mind; you will not fool your subconscious mind. If the anger is there, it is there, how ever well hidden it may be, and you will have to get rid of it, or it will continue to eat away at you, as cancer does. It is very easy to fall into the trap of thinking that all you need to do is to stop stressing yourself in the future. If you do not get rid of your past stress in sufficient measure, you will almost certainly be in trouble. Like the earthquake, you have to get rid of the stress which has built up over the years; that is what made you ill.

Whether you realise it or not, and whether you can contemplate it or not, the real cause for anger is the people who treat you badly now, or who treated you badly in the past. It is they who cause the anger, because they cause difficulties for you, and because, whether you are conscious of it or not, they control your life too much. To some degree, they make you afraid of them, because they are difficult for you, and they stop you enjoying your life as much as you might.

These people might be your parents, from whom you did not get enough love, either because they disciplined you too much, or because, in one way or another, they made too many demands upon you. They may be your husband or wife, or other members of your family, or your immediate companions, from whom you now do not get enough love, or who now make too many demands upon you. They tend to undermine your confidence and your self-esteem; they stress you. If you direct your anger against your illness, when in reality it should be directed against those who make you angry, your real anger will remain, your fear will remain, your sorrow will remain – and your illness will remain.

Even to think of expressing anger against your nearest and dearest can unfortunately be very upsetting. It can make you feel much more guilty than expressing anger against strangers, because it is deeply ingrained in us that really we are supposed to love our nearest and dearest, and certainly we are not supposed to get violently angry with them. It goes against all we have been taught. There may anyway be good reasons why you cannot confront these people face to face. Some, perhaps your parents, may no longer be alive; they may be very old, or they may live far away. In any case, most of us find it upsetting and unpleasant to get very angry in public. If, for whatever reason, it is not possible or appropriate for you to express your anger to these difficult people, face to face in public, you can certainly express it on your own in private. That way only you will know what is happening and nobody will get hurt. It really is vitally important to get rid of this accumulated, suppressed emotion, whether you do it in public, or in private. You will not get rid of it just by thinking about getting rid of it however. All emotion that is freely expressed is expressed through the use of sound and physical movement. As I said before, we roar and shake with anger and we roar and shake with laughter; we moan and shake with fear and we moan and shake with sorrow. A lot of noise is involved and physical action is involved. You are going to have to use sound and physical action to get rid of your suppressed emotion.

It is not so difficult. The easiest way is to shut yourself away in your bedroom, shut the windows and put on the radio so that the neighbours cannot hear, then pick up your pillow and thump hell out of the bed, shouting out your anger against whomever it is who has made your life difficult and stressed you so much in the past, or who is making your life difficult now and is stressing you now. If you prefer not to do this at home, you can go out into the woods, or anywhere else where you can safely be on your own for a short while and let rip with your anger. Tell your difficult people how angry they make you and how angry you are that they have stressed you; call them any names you care to. Really be angry, with a lot of noise and a lot of physical action – really roar and shake with anger.

Acknowledging this anger and getting it out is a very necessary thing to do, not least because it at last really makes you face up to how you have been handling your life. Unless you do face up to this, you will go on accepting things in the same old ways and allowing yourself to be stressed in the same old ways. Your anger – expressed in private – becomes a measure of your determination not to go on stressing yourself in the same old ways. Don't feel ashamed, or guilty, or sorry about what has happened in the past; use your anger to make you determined to control things as you want in the future.

As well as expressing some anger, you are also going to need to have a good cry now and again. Life has not been kind to you; you have not enjoyed it as much as you might have done, and now you have cancer. If you have lost a part of your body through surgery, you most certainly also need to mourn that loss as well. Recognise your sorrow and express your sorrow; don't put on a brave face and suppress it again. Have a good cry when you need to; it is a great stress reliever.

It is also necessary that you acknowledge and express your fear, particularly the fear of your cancer. You have a life-threatening illness and anybody is entitled to find that frightening at first; you are entitled to moan and shake with fear, when you want to. Again, do not try to be brave and hide your fear of cancer, either from yourself, or from your family. It will help your family to express their own fears, for they are probably frightened as well. You may also have had, perhaps for years, a fear of upsetting the difficult people in your life, though you may not always have been conscious of this fear. Get rid of that fear as well, by expressing it. Suppressing emotions has helped to give you cancer. Don't go on doing it.

Since you want to get rid of all this stress as quickly as possible, you should at first spend a few minutes every day giving vent to the emotions you have been suppressing. Don't forget, a lot of noise and a lot of physical action are required. When you have spent those minutes getting rid of some of the backlog, tell yourself, 'there, that's better; I have got rid of the stress for the moment'. That is tremendously important. You have to tell yourself that you have let it go for the moment, you have to believe that you have let it go for the moment, and you really have to feel that you have, whether it is anger, or fear, or sorrow you have been expressing. If you do not do this, the emotion may go on festering inside you for the rest of the day, whereas you need at least a short period when you can be stress free. The emotion will certainly come back again and keep coming back for some time, but, as you gradually get rid of a bit more each day, the effects become less and less. You need to learn to express your emotions much more freely, but you also need to learn to let them go. Remember the arthritics, who express their anger and frustration, but find difficulty in letting it go, and so end up with arthritis. If you express your anger and your other emotions, but do not truly let them go, you may well end up with secondary cancer, if your primary cancer does not get you first.

To help you to feel that you really have got rid of the emotion you have expressed, it is a good thing to end up by having a really good laugh. Laughter triggers off the release of good, healing chemicals into the body, but, in any case, you want to go out of your bedroom with a smile on your face, feeling better, because you have got rid of at least some of the stress which made you ill. Some people are afraid to express anger, because they are afraid that if they keep doing this they will end up a nasty, angry sort of person. It is necessary for you to be aggressive and angry for a time, but you only do this in private, not in public, and, if you always end up by having a good laugh, there is no danger of you turning into a nasty, angry sort of person. Nasty, angry sorts of person are not always laughing.

People do sometimes use laughter, of course, to cover up the stress in their lives. They do not want to acknowledge that they are under stress, or let other people realise that they are under stress, so they laugh to give the appearance that they are happy and not upset. That is another good reason for telling yourself that you have got rid of your stress for the moment, when you laugh, so as really to convince yourself that this is so – at any rate for the moment. Tomorrow you are going to thump your pillow again and get rid of a bit more stress.

It may seem to you at first that to shut yourself away in your bedroom and start shouting with anger, or crying, or moaning with fear, are very childish and ridiculous things to do. It may feel like that the first time you do it; you may feel that you ought to pull yourself together and act like a grown up. These are natural enough feelings, because mum and dad were continually telling us to sit up, shut up, and behave ourselves, when we were kids, and we therefore tend to feel guilty and even self indulgent if, for a time, we do disobey and indulge ourselves in this way.

The essential thing to remember is that you became ill because you were too stressed and that you have therefore got to be determined to de-stress yourself; you want to give yourself the best chance of recovery you possibly can. Never mind therefore, if at first, it all sounds a bit childish and ridiculous, never mind if, at first, it all feels a bit childish and ridiculous; do it; get rid of the stress. Express the emotions, let them go, and de-stress yourself. There are times when a spade should be called a spade. If anybody, or everybody, always expects you to do what they want, they are treating you as the next best thing to a doormat, however surprised they might be to have this pointed out to them. If your conscious mind does not pick up the message that you are being treated as the next best thing to a doormat, your subconscious mind certainly will. It is a message which would eat away at anyone's self esteem and it is a form of treatment which fully justifies your anger. Thumping your pillow is a simple and safe way to express your anger and a simple and safe way to express your determination not to go on accepting any longer that you must go on accepting stress in your life without protest.

If you express your anger in private, nobody else need know and nobody will get hurt. If, however, you do wish to express your anger face to face with your difficult person or persons, and tell them exactly what you think about them, do so. The choice is yours. Clearly, there is the risk attached to this that this confrontation may lead to a break up of the relationship. Sadly, in some cases, this is what may really be necessary. Better a live, but divorced wife or husband, seeking happiness elsewhere, than a dead wife or husband who continued an impossibly stressful relationship for too long.

'Divorce', temporary or permanent, may also sometimes be appropriate between you and other members of your family, if that is what it takes to keep you alive. Do not feel guilty about it. It may just help those concerned to treat you a little better and be a little less difficult in the future. Recognition of what has really been going on in the past can bring reconciliation. Recognition can come on all sides that all of us are products of our upbringing, and, with this, can come forgiveness.

People sometimes fear, that, if they start to express anger against their parents, even if they do this in private, they may end up hating their parents. If it was your parents who gave you a hard time, you need to get this anger out, because it will go on eating away at you otherwise. If you do keep getting it out every day and letting it go, inevitably you will eventually get rid of it all and one day, when you pick up your pillow, you will find that you truly do not feel anger any more; you have got rid of it all. You may still feel some sadness about the situation, but there is no anger left. If you want to, and if you think it will make you feel better – and it probably will – say to yourself then, "ok mum and dad; I do not like the way you brought me up, because it helped to make me ill, but I have got rid of the anger now, so here's a big hug, because I suppose that in many ways it was not entirely your fault; you only brought me up in the sort of ways in which you were brought up by your parents". The same can apply just as well with other people in your life who have been difficult for you. If you get rid of the anger, either you can forgive them, or you can get to the point where you feel you just can't be bothered with them any more – there is no anger left and there is no stress left. Forgiveness, or indifference, it does not really matter what the end result is, you have got rid of this stress from your life.

It is only through getting your anger out and letting it go that you will be able truly to forgive people, if that is what you want to do. You will not truly be able to forgive them in any other way. If you try to do it by thinking only loving and forgiving thoughts, or by thinking that other people may need to express their anger, but you don't, your suppressed anger will almost certainly remain, suppressed inside you, eating away at you. Once again, it may be easy to fool your conscious mind; it is not easy to fool your subconscious.

If you have not expressed your emotions freely for years, the first burst of real emotion may feel frightening, because it is so violent. Your reaction may be to clamp down hastily on the safety valve again and bottle it up once more. This merely increases the pressure in the boiler again and makes you feel more depressed, so resist the temptation. If you had been brought up to use the safety valve properly in the past to release a little emotion each time you felt emotion, you would not now have such a backlog to get rid of. All you are doing now – in private – is catching up as quickly as possible on lost time.

Make sure that you do express all your emotions, anger,

fear, sorrow and joy. It is easy to fall into the trap of only expressing the one which seems to come up most easily. Women, who have been taught that it is acceptable for them to cry, but not acceptable for them to get angry, can end up spending a lot of time crying and no time being angry. Men, who have been taught that it is acceptable for them sometimes to be angry, but not acceptable for them to cry, can end up never crying.

You will find that on some days not all the emotions need to come out, or you may find on some days that one emotion is much stronger than the others; we are not always the same each day. Anger is certainly the principal emotion you need to express, but it is important to give yourself the chance, every day, to express all the emotions, to see what does want to come out. Don't run the risk of continuing to suppress emotions by not bothering to see what there is to be expressed.

If it really feels very strange and uncomfortable at first to express your emotions violently, it may help you to ham it up a bit to begin with. Pretend that you are the famous actor or actress rehearsing for a play. You have to rehearse these very emotional parts, the very angry person, the extremely frightened person, the deeply sorrowful person, the rumbustiously happy person. The great actor was once asked to what he attributed his success as an actor. "Sincerity, sincerity", he replied; "get them to believe that and they will believe anything". It makes a good story, but, of course, it is absolutely true. As great actors and actresses study and learn their parts, they come to feel that they are the persons they have to portray. They get right under the skin of their character and they become that character, rather than themselves. They do use total sincerity in their 'acting'. That is what you have to do. When you are really living the part, rather than acting it, your suppressed emotions will flow freely and you will gradually get rid of that pile of straw that accumulated on your back.

As well as deliberately expressing some anger, and possibly other emotions, in whatever way you want to, it is important to reinforce this by always trying to keep a check on yourself at any time. If you do find that you are getting up-tight during the day, it is easy just to take a slightly deeper breath, just tense up a little more – maybe clench your fists, or grit your teeth slightly – and then let your breath out and release the tension. Nobody else need notice or be aware; you can do it quickly and without attracting attention. If you are on your own and can give a good shout to get rid of the tension and stress, so much the better. Do keep checking on yourself very consciously. It has become an unconscious habit to stress yourself and now you have to make it a very conscious habit to de-stress yourself. If you really get upset and angry, when you are with others, but it is not possible or appropriate to express your emotion there and then in public, save it up until you are somewhere in private, where you can express it and let it go; don't forget about it and suppress it – and don't forget to smile when you have let it go, to tell yourself that you have let it go, and to feel that you have let it go. Releasing tension and stress for yourself in these ways is very liberating; it frees you from the inhibiting restraints of the past; it is something you should do for the rest of your life. You, in particular, never want to get into the habit again of suppressing emotion.

In the 1960's, the so-called encounter groups became popular in the United States and later in other countries. Groups met together and individuals were encouraged to give violent vent to their emotions in front of their fellows in the group. Some found this very therapeutic, and no doubt some who attend encounter groups today also find it so. Most of us probably would not wish to emote in this way in public. There is no need to. The same effect can be achieved equally well on your own and in the privacy of your home, where there is nobody else to embarrass you and nobody else to get hurt.

8

How to Stop Putting Straw onto your Back

Releasing and letting go of stress, whenever you start to feel it, is the first step which helps you to stop piling straw onto your back. What you must also learn is how to deal more appropriately with the people who cause you difficulties, either because they aggressively demand too much of you, or because you feel it is your duty continually to look after their interests, rather than your own. You have to learn not to accept and submit to this sort of situation. This does not mean that you have to become aggressive towards these people. Being aggressive in public towards others is distasteful to most of us and is anyway unnecessary. Certainly you have to be very aggressive in getting rid of the pile of straw which is already on your back, but this you do in private, not in public, and you end up by letting go of your aggression and having a good laugh to ensure that you have let it go.

To stop putting straw onto your back, you have to become assertive, not aggressive, with your difficult people. Being assertive means saying clearly what it is you feel and want. It means saying, 'yes, I hear what you say and I understand what you feel and want; however, what I feel and what I want . . .'. Assertiveness is therefore about honest communication. It is not about winning the point at issue. You may not win the point, but you will have expressed your feelings and your wants, and not suppressed them, and this is the vital point. It is precisely because we often cannot say what we feel and what we want to certain people, that, consciously or subconsciously, we feel anger. Our inability to express what we feel and what we want can not only make us angry, it can make us sad and depressed that we cannot enjoy our lives more. We are afraid of upsetting others and they are more in control of our lives than we are.

The only effective way to change the way someone habitually acts towards you is to change the way in which you habitually react towards them. If you usually say yes, you have to start saying no. At first the other person may not notice that you are saying no, and may continue to act as if you were still saying yes, because they are used to you always saying yes. If you continue to say no, however, and act accordingly, they will begin to realise that you are saying no and that you mean no, and they will be forced to treat you and the situation differently.

Once again, it is a question of practising in private first, before you get on to the real thing. You have to learn to play this new part and you need to learn the new lines and the new movements. You can rehearse on your own, or with a sympathetic friend, or you can go to a local assertiveness training group. It is perfectly easy to rehearse on your own. It can help to start by putting an empty chair in front of you and imagining that the person you find difficult is sitting in the chair. Then go back over a recent conversation with them, when you gave in to what they wanted, rather than stuck out for what you wanted. Practise the sort of conversation you would like to have had with this person, in which you would have told them exactly what it was you wanted without difficulty. You may find at first that you lose your temper and start telling the person just what you think of them. That is all right; you are just shedding a bit more straw from your back. When you have let off steam, don't forget to tell yourself that you have let your anger go again for the moment, and then have a good laugh. Then start again and have the assertive conversation you wish to have with your person. Keep practising until you get it right.

Almost inevitably, of course, a real live conversation with your difficult person will at first not go exactly as you rehearsed it; these things rarely do, but there is a technique you can use, which will help you. If you remember the old 78 rpm records, you will remember how, when they got scratched, the needle would get stuck in a groove and the record would go on repeating the same little bit of music over and over again. When your difficult person tries to ride roughshod over what you have said, just keep on like the scratched record, repeating, "yes, I hear what you say, but, I repeat, what I feel and what I want is . . .'. That is all you need to say and keep repeating. Keep it as simple as that. Don't try to give reasons, or elaborate on why you do or don't want something, or you will find yourself getting into an argument. Don't go on too long, however, if your difficult person refuses to hear what you are saying. Get up and go and then come back to the point at some later time. Tell them, "I have told you what I feel and what I want", and then go. If you keep on and on trying to make your point, they may well wear you down and you may end up giving in to them again. They have had a lot of practice at doing this and they are very good at it. You will end up feeling angry, frustrated, confused and tired, because these people easily drain you of energy. Even when you only make your point two or three times and then go, you may still find that you feel angry. That is quite understandable and natural. Go and thump your pillow, express your anger and let it go; don't bottle it up and suppress it. As you start to make progress with your difficult persons, you will find that you don't get so angry, because they are starting to acknowledge you and what you feel and want. You are getting back into control of your life.

If your difficulty is that you are always looking after everyone else, rather than that you have difficulty with one or two particular people, you still have to practise saying no, rather than yes. Again, practise by going back over recent situations, when you have said yes, when you wanted to, or ought to have said no. Imagine how the conversation might have gone. There are a number of quite acceptable ways of saying no: I shall not have the time; I prefer to do something else; I am doing something else; or just plain, no, I do not want to. When you are assertive, the message that your mind sends to your body is 'relax, there is no danger if I say no; this is not a real dinosaur which will eat me up if I say no; it is only a paper dinosaur; there is no real danger'. If you convince your body that you really mean what you say, the adrenalin will cease to flow, your body will get back into chemical balance again, and the physical tension will leave your body.

Sadly, some spouses find it difficult to face up to the fact that their partner has cancer, perhaps through fear, and they try to leave their partner to cope alone. This is another occasion for assertiveness and for telling the spouse how helpful it would be to have their support, so that both of you might work together as the team you should be. If this should happen to you, it would be a good idea, first of all, to thump your pillow and get rid of your anger in private, but then you must keep on insisting quietly and assertively on your right to have your spouse's support. It is your right and you are entitled to insist upon it; do not go on accepting this difficult situation; it is stressful for you. Tell your spouse how much it stresses you not to have their help and that you need to get stress out of your life, if you are to get better.

The important thing with difficult people is not to lose your temper. If you lose your temper and become aggressive, the situation deteriorates rapidly into a slanging match, which increases the bad feelings between you and makes life even more difficult. You vent your anger in private. In public, you keep your temper and are assertive, not aggressive. Look on assertiveness as the mid-point on the scale which runs from extreme aggressiveness at one end of the scale, to extreme submissiveness at the other end of the scale. The more you can keep the scales in balance, with the pointer on the scale near to the mid-point of assertiveness, without violent fluctuations towards aggressiveness, or submissiveness, the more balanced and enjoyable your life will be; you will be in control of your emotions, rather than them being in control of you. Aggressiveness and submissiveness help you to pile straw onto your back. Assertiveness helps you to stop piling straw onto your back.

Assertiveness does require practice, but the more you practise it, the better you will become at it. Don't start off by confronting your difficult people with the really big and important issues. Start off with minor things and be as assertive as you can with these. It is not so important if things do not go so well with these. Leave the important issues until later, when you have become more used to speaking and acting assertively and feel more confident about getting your points across.

Inevitably at first you will get it wrong sometimes and still say yes, when you ought to say no. There are two things you can do. Either go back to the person concerned and say that, having thought it over, you have decided after all that you do not want to do whatever it was. Stick to your position assertively, without losing your temper. Alternatively, if this is not possible, just write off your mistake to experience. Tell yourself, ok, so I got it wrong this time; next time I will be more careful. That is being assertive with yourself. Don't get angry with yourself; that is being aggressive with yourself, which you don't want to be on this sort of occasion. It is bad enough that you are now going to have to do something you don't really want to do; don't kick yourself as well.

Body language can be important in dealing assertively with others, and you may find it helpful to practise being assertive in front of a mirror. You need to be as relaxed as possible, so you need to be breathing in a calm, relaxed manner. Then you just need to stand or sit still and upright, look the other person in the eye and say what it is you want to say clearly and directly. Hunching up, moving about, and dropping the eyes are all signs of nervousness and submissiveness.

As you learn to be more assertive and to communicate clearly what you want, you will become more at ease with yourself and find that you have a greater respect for yourself, because now you are not allowing your life to be controlled by others. You are your own person. Trying to please everyone else in life is merely a subconscious way of trying to buy their love. To feel that you must buy everyone else's love is hardly good for your sense of self-esteem. You cannot be your own person when you continually have to be subservient to others in this way. Your sense of self-esteem is tremendously important. If you do not have it in sufficient measure, life gets very depressing and life can even cease to have any real meaning or worth for you. None of us has a perfect upbringing and in consequence none of us is perfect – nor ever will be. When you have a real sense of self-esteem, however, you are at ease with yourself and it is easy to live with the fact that you are not perfect. You can accept yourself as you are, warts and all. It is no longer so important if you are wrong on occasion; so is everybody else on occasion, including all those people you previously found so difficult. It is no longer so important to have the approval of others, when you have self-esteem. When you are in control of your life, others do not easily put you down and you do not feel the need to put others down. You are a more balanced person.

Ideally, the difficult people in your life should also receive counselling, to teach them to be less demanding on you. This is unlikely to happen, but, as you learn to be assertive, you will find that they do treat you differently and that they do become less difficult, because your changed way of dealing with them does not allow them to treat you in their old difficult style.

Let me emphasise again that it can be dangerous to think that all your troubles will be solved if you just learn to be assertive and that you do not need to thump your pillow as well. Being assertive sounds much more grown up than thumping your pillow, which is partly why it can appeal more. If you have thumped your pillow first, however, you will have got rid of some of your anger and you will find it easier to be assertive without losing your temper. Even more important, however, is that the more stress, conscious and subconscious, you get out of your life, the better chance you have of recovering from your illness.

It is through the actual experience of expressing yourself freely that you come to learn that it is not really dangerous to do this; you can let go of your fear; the sky does not fall in on you and the world does not come to an end. You can learn that, if you are honest with other people, it is often easier for them to be honest with you. Both sides end up knowing where the other stands and the relationship becomes an easier one. When you are afraid to speak your mind, maybe because you think you must keep the peace, it is as if you are hiding behind a facade, or playing a role which is not really you.

It is because it can feel frightening to start expressing yourself freely that it can be so helpful to start practising this in private, before you attempt too much in public. As you do start to feel able to express yourself more freely, it becomes a process of self-discovery, as you stop having to play false roles and start to become the person you really are. It is a process of growth and development, maybe a bit scary at first, but exciting and fulfilling. Life should be a process of growth and development, if we are to fulfill ourselves and be our own person. We too should blossom as the rose.

9

A Few Things to Beware of

Some healers do not like facing up to the existence of anger as a human emotion, just like some patients. They prefer to pretend that it does not, or should not exist. In some healing circles, more importance seems sometimes to be attached to having patients transcend the mundane things of this world, with the emphasis on love, spirituality, and saving patients' souls, rather than their lives. Healing seems to become limited to some rather ill-defined opening up of patients' spiritual awareness, with the implication that, if you reach this desirable state, it is then quite all right for you to die, because you have been 'healed'.

I believe that patients come along because they wish to have their lives saved. We are body, mind and spirit, and holistic healing will be interested in healing patients in all three, not just in healing them in spirit. To limit healing to the spiritual aspects of our humanity is to under-value and degrade that humanity. Certainly, if patients are to die – and some will – it is preferable that they die spiritually at peace. If patients are not to die – and I believe that many more might be taught to survive – it is necessary to remove physical, mental and spiritual stress from their lives, not just spiritual stress.

This desire to save souls is sometimes reflected in the 'love is all you need' approach. If you have been told, and therefore believe, that it is wrong to give vent to your emotions, and perhaps particularly to your anger, it is going to be very hard for you to do this. It will feel wrong and, quite naturally, it will make you feel guilty, because you are disobeying mum and dad. An easy way out may seem to be that offered by some therapists, to smother everything with love. If only you were full of love, you may think – and you may be told – you would somehow get rid of all those nasty, baser emotions, which seem to lurk beneath the surface. Love and spirituality, in sufficiently large spoonfuls, is really all you need, you may be told – and you may come to believe. Anger and fear and sorrow are often thought of as negative emotions, with love or joy as the only positive emotion. We need to understand that our ability to express anger, fear and sorrow, as well as joy, provides the absolutely essential safety valve we need to deal with excessive stress in our lives. Certainly there are appropriate and inappropriate ways and times in which to express our emotions, but express them we must – all of them – if we are to get rid of the stress in our lives. The therapist who tries to teach you that all will be solved by love and spirituality, does you no service. This merely encourages you to go on suppressing emotions, which you will have been suppressing probably over a long period of time, and which will have been a major factor in making you ill. If you go on suppressing these emotions, you may die.

Religion is sometimes invoked in the cause of love and spirituality and can therefore sometimes seem to be the culprit, for it seems to tell us that we must always seek to become better, to strive towards perfection. Surely, you may tell yourself, to be a perfect human being means to be full of love and spirituality, to the exclusion of all else. There are examples in the Bible, however, when Christ showed anger, grief and fear – his anger at the money-lenders in the temple, his grief at the news of Lazarus' death, his fear of his own impending death. We do not seem to regard this expression of emotions as sinful, or in any way unwarranted. Christ lived amongst us as a human being and showed and expressed these human emotions in appropriate fashion and at appropriate times. We may certainly do the same throughout our human lives; we are not machines; we need to feel and express our human emotions, if we are to be fully human.

The exhortation that we should turn the other cheek can also lead to misunderstanding. It should not make you think that sublimating your anger will dispose of it. If God is the all seeing God we are told He is, He will be well aware that your anger and resentment still exist in your subconscious, if you have not expressed and got rid of them. By all means turn the other cheek in public, but then express and get rid of your anger and resentment in private. Then both you and God will know that you have truly forgiven your neighbour.

Religion should also not be used to make you fall into the trap of thinking that your cancer is some form of devil to be cast out in the name of religion. The cancer is a growth, which you must help and encourage your immune system to destroy. It is a part of your body which has gone wrong, because of the stress you have been under. It is not a devil from the nether regions.

Some may encourage you to hand all your problems to God, in the pious hope that He will take your cancer away from you. This may sound like a good idea, but, in fact it is merely a way of absolving yourself from having to face up to your difficulties and from having to deal with them. It continues the too accepting and submissive approach, which is at the root of the illness. Any cancer patients who are encouraged to hand all their problems to God are being encouraged not to fight their illness as actively as they might and they are, therefore, the less likely to survive.

We do need a great deal of love in our lives and we do not always get it. Our religion, if we understand it, offers us abundant love, but also says that we should channel and use our emotions, not suppress them. It is the balanced teaching we should also get from our parents, but sometimes do not.

10

Positive Self-healing through Visualisation

Starting to get rid of the past mental stress in your life and seeing that you do not stress yourself mentally in the future will begin to give your body the stress-free conditions it needs to heal itself. Now you need to give your body some active encouragement to heal itself. This you can do through what has come to be called visualisation, which is just another word for the act of using your imagination. To use visualisation effectively, and also to practise meditation, which I will discuss later, you need to be as physically relaxed as possible. At this point therefore, I want to digress on to the importance of learning to breathe in a truly relaxed way.

Breathing may not strike you as being very important; after all, we breathe all the time, without thinking about it. Slow, relaxed breathing, however, is the basis of all physical relaxation and it is vital to good health. Most of us breathe very shallowly and we tend to breathe only in the top of the chest, so that we do not have enough oxygen circulating through our bodies. If you are intent on something such as writing, or reading, you are under slight stress. If you stop to check, you may find that you have almost stopped breathing. It is impossible to be mentally or physically up-tight if you are breathing in a slow relaxed fashion.

When you exert yourself, by running down the road for instance, it is easy to see the chest rising and falling. We need to do some of this chest breathing periodically, not least because we get a great deal of tension in the chest area, and in the area of the neck and shoulders, and we need to keep these areas as free and relaxed as possible. We also need to take some fairly vigorous exercise two or three times a week. In relaxed breathing, however, it is the stomach which should be moving rather more than the chest. You have a sheet of muscle, called the diaphragm, which goes right across the body, separating the chest cavity from the stomach cavity. In relaxed breathing when you breathe in, the air going into your lungs presses down on your diaphragm and this pushes out the stomach slightly. When you breathe out, your stomach moves in again.

The best way to practise this stomach breathing is to do it lying down. Lie on your back, just move your arms and legs and your head a little, to make sure you are as relaxed as you can be to start with, then place your hands on your stomach, just below the ribs, and start to breathe away, gradually slowing your breathing right down. Breathe in slowly, then pause for a second, before breathing out slowly. Another slight pause, then breathe in again slowly. When you breathe out, take a little longer over it than when you breathe in; it is more relaxing that way. If you find this way of breathing difficult, and some people do at first, start by holding your breath, then pull your stomach in and push it out by contracting and then releasing your stomach muscles. Repeat this, but this time, as you push your stomach out, breathe in; then as you pull your stomach in, breathe out. At first it may seem as if you are doing things the wrong way round, but practise it until it feels natural to breathe in this way. The stomach is more or less the centre of the body and stomach breathing will also help you to feel 'centred' and more balanced in your body. Think of it in this way too, as well as of it being the best way to be relaxed.

As you gradually learn to breathe in this slow, easy, relaxed way, you will find that you really are becoming more and more relaxed. Breathing in this way slows down your heart and pulse rates and helps to lower your blood pressure. It is also a very helpful way of getting to sleep, but it is something you should practise all the time, at any odd moment of the day, until it does become a natural habit for you. Practise it whilst you are eating; it helps the digestion and therefore helps your body to absorb the vitamins and minerals from your food. Practise it in the car, practise it walking down the street, practise it whilst you are watching the television. Practise it at home and at work, whenever and wherever you can. It may seem unimportant; it is actually vitally important.

Some use biofeedback machines, such as skin resistance meters, to learn to relax and these can be useful, because they give a physical indication of how relaxed you are. Unfortunately, those who are very tense often find they are of no help, because they are so tense that they cannot get the indicator needle to move. They need to be taught to breathe properly to help them to relax, and then of course they do not need a biofeedback machine anyway.

There are other physical stress factors besides breathing, and I will discuss these later. Let us return to visualisation. Many sports people use visualisation to help them play their sport better. You have first of all to study and understand the technique of your game; you have to know how to perform the particular golf shot for instance. Then you practise it in your mind, imagining yourself making the shot perfectly, time after time. When you actually stand in front of the golf ball, about to make the shot, you relax physically, imagine yourself making the shot perfectly, and then carry out the shot. The more time you have spent beforehand visualising yourself making the shot perfectly, the more likely you are to make the shot perfectly. If you get up-tight physically or mentally – in other words, if you start to feel that you may not be able to make the shot – you stand a much higher chance of making a mess of the shot. Your mind tells your body that there is danger and your body becomes physically tense. Imagining that you are going to make the shot well helps to overcome the fear that you will not be able to make the shot well, because your mind is occupied with success, rather than the possibility of failure. You are sending the message to your body, relax, there's no danger – which is a nice healing message for your golf and helps to make your sick golf better.

There is a simple, general visualisation exercise, which you can practise at any time for a few moments, as a means of reminding yourself to keep your stress levels down. You can even do it walking down the road, but keep your eyes open if you do it then. It is an easy way to start practising visualisation. First get yourself relaxed and slow your breathing right down. Then, as you breathe in, imagine – and tell yourself – that you are drawing healing right up through your body; remember that your body knows how to heal itself and wants to heal itself. Starting from your toes and your fingers, imagine the healing flowing up through your legs and arms, right up to the top of your head. Try to feel a nice warm glow moving up through you, through every part of your body, so that every part of your body feels free and relaxed. As you breathe out, imagine – and tell yourself – that all the surplus, stressful tension in your body is draining out through your body and out through your toes and your fingers. You need some tension in your muscles, other-wise you would collapse in a heap, so it is only the surplus tension you breathe out. It may help you to imagine waves flowing in and out of your body, like waves on a sea shore. You want to feel that your body is completely cleansed and that there are no tension blockages any-where. You want to feel that the energy flows freely through your body.

If you have difficulty imagining this idea of flow from your toes to the top of your head, try a slightly different variation. As you breathe in, imagine yourself as a sort of balloon and feel yourself expanding slightly as you breathe the healing into yourself. As you breathe out the unnecessary tension, imagine yourself deflating slightly.

Whichever way you choose, watch out for tension around
your eyes, jaw and throat, where it builds up again easily,
especially if you are 'talking' to yourself, telling yourself to
relax.

Some healers say that it is unnecessary to tell the body
to heal itself, because it knows how to and will, if it is
given stress-free conditions. Whilst this is true, I believe
that it is very important for you to tell it what you want it
to do, whilst you are visualising it doing this, because this
involves you very much more directly and positively in
your own healing. Our bodies do have immense self-
healing powers, but the more you consciously send healing messages to your body, the more you will build up
your confidence in your body's powers and the more you
will begin to know that you can and do control your body.
Your body does get the message, if you send the message
often enough. Subconsciously, you sent stress messages to
your body and eventually you became ill. Now, consciously send healing messages, until your body does get
the new message. You want to speed up the healing
process as much as you can.

Visualisation can obviously be used for any specific part
of the body, which needs particular attention. You can
also go on to use much more specific imagery, if you want
to, rather than the general imagery I have just described.
To give some examples, the person with an ulcer might
imagine warm, healing oil flowing through their stomach,
soothing the ulcerated area. The person with joints swol-
len with arthritis might imagine that the swellings were
solidified sugar and that hot tea flowing through them
was dissolving the swellings. The person with a cataract
might imagine that the cataract was made of gelatine and
that they were pouring hot water onto the gelatine to melt
it. The person with multiple sclerosis could imagine thin
optical fibres replacing the parts of their nerves which had
become scarred, so that the brain could still flash its
'lighted' messages successfully right throughout the body.
This imagery could also be used by cancer patients, who

have had part of their lymphatic systems removed by surgery, to get the body to repair and find new ways round the damaged areas. Our bodies will try to adapt to new conditions as far as they possibly can and they can often do much more in this way than we believe.

If you have got cancer, you can also use a wide variety of images to imagine your body being cleansed of cancer cells and the cancerous tumours being dissolved or disposed of in some way. The most straightforward way perhaps is to imagine the white blood cells, which are the cells which fight off infections in the body, attacking and destroying the cancer cells; maybe the white blood cells could be white knights on white horses. You may like to imagine a white light flooding through your body, God's light if you like, or maybe you could have a white laser beam seeking out and destroying the cancer cells.

Another more specific image for cancer would be to have a large golden eagle flying overhead in your body, keeping a close, eagle-eyed watch for any cancer cells stirring below and swooping down to destroy them, wherever they appeared. You can have herds of cattle, or geese, moving round your body, twenty-four hours a day, eating up any cancer cells they find. You can have armies of little soldiers marching round your body, killing off cancer cells. If you are a keen gardener, you can go round the garden of your body, digging out cancer cells, roots and all. You can have fish swimming round your body, gobbling up cancer cells. You can scrub your inside clean with a hard scrubbing brush, or put your body cells through a washing machine to clean them up daily. You can imagine yourself standing under a shower, or a waterfall, with the water flowing right through every cell of your body, washing the cancer cells out of you. There are many different ways of imagining cancer cells being destroyed.

If you have leukaemia, it is your white blood cells which are cancerous and you will need to direct your imagery towards getting your white cells better initially. One of my patients with leukaemia had had all his white blood cells knocked out by chemotherapy and was in hospital, being kept 'fit' by antibiotics, whilst waiting for his white blood cell count to rise again, hopefully with good, healthy white cells. His blood count would not rise, so I suggested to him that he imagine a white blood cell factory in his body, which would now start to produce white blood cells for him. There would be a unit in the factory to put into each white cell the 'x' factor it needed to be an effective cell, and there would be an inspection unit at the factory gate to ensure that every cell was one hundred percent perfect and that any sub-standard cells were destroyed and not allowed to leave the factory. The patient started this visualisation and within a few days his white blood cell count shot up and there was no sign of cancer. It is quite possible to argue that this would have happened anyway, and maybe it would have done. The patient believed that the visualisation had helped; it most certainly seemed to help to increase markedly his confidence in his ability to influence his own recovery and that alone is tremendously important. Interestingly, the patient was an actor and good visualisation is akin to acting – sincerity, once again. The more sincerity you put into your visualisation and the more you believe that it can and will work, the more likely it is to work. Your body gets the message. You could of course also use this 'factory' type of imagery to increase your red blood cell and platelet counts, if these are also low as a result of your leukaemia.

Visualisation can also be used for pain control. Try to visualise your pain; how big is it? what shape is it? what colour is it? Now see if you can soften the colour to a softer pastel shade. Then see if you can place your hands on it and stroke it and soothe it, gently making it a little smaller; give it some tender loving care. Another way you might find helpful is to use the wave imagery, imagining waves flowing through the pain area, as you breathe in and out, cooling and soothing the area.

Pain can become worse if we worry about it, so although it has nothing to do directly with visualisation, it may help you to do anything which will help to distract you for a time, becoming absorbed in a book, or a play, or in music, or singing, or painting, or whatever it may be. It is known that laughter triggers off the release of endorphins in the body, which help to relieve pain, so anything which really helps you to laugh can also be very helpful. Get some amusing books or videos out of the library, watch all the comedians on the television, or listen to them on the radio, go to comedy plays and films. The more you can laugh and cheer yourself up, the better you will feel for a while. Another way to tackle pain is by using coffee enemas and I will discuss this in Chapter 14.

Visualisation can also be helpful, if you are having radiotherapy or chemotherapy, because it can help to lessen the side effects. If you are having radiotherapy, you might imagine that the rays are healing rays, God's healing rays if you like, which are going to kill off the cancer cells, but strengthen your normal cells, so that they are not harmed and not burned. During the weeks you are having radiotherapy, you could also imagine periodically that the area being treated is being bathed with cooling, healing oils or ointment, so as to prevent it burning. Radiotherapy continues its effects after you finish the treatment, so don't stop your visualisation when you stop your treatment; side effects can still start to occur a week or two later.

Similarly with chemotherapy, you can imagine that the drugs are healing substances, which will only kill off the cancer cells they find anywhere in your body, but will strengthen and help your normal cells. You might imagine that you have a special little computer somewhere in your body, which automatically programmes the chemotherapy drugs, so that they only attack cancer cells, but at the same time release a special healing fluid for all your other cells. If your chemotherapy goes on for several hours, don't try to practise visualisation the whole time. You won't manage to do it successfully and it gets boring anyway. Do it for a few minutes every hour, but do it then with real conviction.

Radiotherapy and chemotherapy can gradually make you feel tired and lacking in energy, as the treatment progresses. Use visualisation to help yourself. You can imagine that your hands and feet are five-pin electric plugs, which you plug into the universal energy system of Creation; energy really is all around us in trees and plants and birds and animals, in the earth and the sun and the stars. As you breathe in, draw energy into your body through your fingers and toes from the energy all around you. As you breathe out, imagine the energy circulating all round your body; do not breathe it out again, because you want it to build up in your body and recharge your batteries. Plug yourself into the system several times a day and keep topping yourself up. Tell yourself how full of energy you are, when you have topped yourself up, and feel the energy flowing through you.

Hair loss is sometimes another unfortunate side effect of chemotherapy. One lady told me that, when she was having chemotherapy, she used to visualise that all the hairs of her head were tied to her head with tight knots just below her scalp. Her hair did not fall out, though to be fair, not every combination of chemotherapy drugs makes the hair fall out. A nice story though and well worth a try if you are having the sort of chemotherapy which does cause hair loss.

I think the example of visualisation I like best is of the lady who visualised herself as bionic woman throughout the time she was having chemotherapy. Both she and her consultant were surprised by how much energy she had all the time and by how well she did – well, if you were bionic woman, I suppose you would, wouldn't you? When she stopped her chemotherapy, she stopped doing her visualisation and over the next few months she gradually got more and more tired. It took her some time to realise why; she had stopped being bionic woman. She went back to her visualisation and got back her drive and her energy again.

It is always best if you yourself choose whatever imagery you want to use in visualisation, because then it is much more likely to work for you. What is important, when you are using it to destroy cancer cells, is that the destroying imagery should be visualised as being much stronger than the cancer cells it is attacking. You should imagine the cancer cells as being grey and weak, never, for instance, as red or black, which are strong colours, and don't imagine them as being solid and hard. It is little use imagining the cancer to be a block of stone, at which you are chipping away with a hammer and cold chisel – the block of stone is almost certainly going to win. The imagery you use has to be sufficiently aggressive for it to have a real chance of working and for you to believe that it has a real chance of working.

There is a school of thought which says that, since your cancer cells are part of you, you should not use aggressive imagery in visualisation, since this is to be aggressive against yourself. I agree that we need to love ourselves and that some of us may need to learn to love ourselves more; self-esteem is a most important factor in good health. However, to ask us to love something, even within our own bodies, which may kill us, is to ask too much of us I believe. Our immune systems, which we may certainly love and encourage, work by attacking and rejecting what they see as foreign intruders in our bodies. That is why those having organ transplants have to be given immuno-suppressive drugs, to try to prevent their immune systems rejecting the transplanted organ. To try to love your cancer cells back into good cells, when your immune system wishes to reject and destroy them, is therefore to try to work against your own immune system, which does not sound like a good idea.

Whatever type of visualisation you decide to do, it is essential that you practise it regularly. It is highly unlikely to do any good if you practise it half-heartedly, or if you only practise it once a fortnight, when you happen to remember it. It may help to start off by doing it for only three or four minutes at a time, so as to try to do it really well, with real conviction; quality is very necessary. Try to do it a number of times during the day. Once you feel you are doing it well, try to do it for longer, but cut down the number of times you do it a little. Aim to do it eventually for at least fifteen to twenty minutes at a time and aim to do this at least twice, and preferably three times a day.

We can all visualise to some extent; if you can remember what your family look like, you can visualise. If you really do have difficulty in visualising internal images, however, it may help to start by concentrating on getting to be aware of feelings in your body. Try an exercise first of all with your hands. Get relaxed and close your eyes. Put your hands on your thighs and then try to imagine that you can feel them gradually getting warmer and heavier. Think of the sun shining on them, or think of them being in hot water. The hands are the best part of the body to start with, because we use the hands all the time for touching and handling things and we can be more easily aware of feelings in them. Once you can make your hands feel warm and heavy, try your feet, then gradually extend the feeling of warmth and heaviness right up through your body. One point of the exercise is to help to make you become more aware of your body, so that at any time during the day you can become aware of any physical tension and can learn to release it. You may also find, however, that when you have practised this sort of exercise for a bit, it becomes easier for you to use the normal type of visualisation, precisely because you are more aware of your body and what can and does go on in it.

Visualisation involves you directly and positively in your own healing, so it is very important to keep practising it regularly, every day. If you find your attention wandering, as it will from time to time, just bring it gently back to the visualisation again. Your concentration will gradually improve as you keep practising. Keep things relatively simple. The body does know how to heal itself, so, although it helps to tell it what to do, because this gets you involved in your healing, there is no need to give your body complicated instructions in what to do. If you go into too much detail, you may get something slightly wrong. You do not need to know exactly how your body works and simple ideas are quite sufficient for visualisation. Trust your body to get the details right.

When your body is functioning efficiently and you are healthy, it is as if your body is functioning according to an original blueprint of how it should function. Use your visualisation therefore to imagine your white blood cells, in whatever form you choose, flooding in, surrounding, destroying and flushing away any abnormal, cancerous cells that there may be in your body. Your cancer cells are obviously abnormal cells, because they would not be in the blueprint of a normal, healthy body. With the abnormal cells out of the way, normal cells can take over again and your body can regenerate itself, with the red blood cells bringing oxygen and nourishment back to the whole area. Your body gets back to its original, healthy blueprint; you heal yourself. As I said before, if you have leukaemia, you will have to adapt the imagery to suit your own particular circumstances, but here too keep to the general idea of getting your body back to its healthy blueprint. Your visualisation will almost certainly be more effective, if you keep to basic, simple concepts; don't over complicate things.

Visualisation is important above all because it harnesses the immense power of the human mind to the immense self-healing power of the human body. It will help you to build up your confidence in your body's ability to heal itself and it will help to strengthen your determination to fight and beat your cancer. It is the fighters who almost always do best.

11

Relaxation through Meditation

Meditation is another excellent relaxation technique you should use to help to de-stress yourself. If you have never come across it before, the idea of meditating may sound a bit way out, but there is nothing strange or complicated about it. Meditation can be carried out on your own, or in a group. As with visualisation, with which it can have links, it is first necessary to be as physically relaxed as possible. There is no need to sit in an advanced yoga position, though do, if you are into yoga and it helps you to do so. You can do it sitting in an armchair, or lying down, if you prefer. Some like to have the spine upright; again, it is not absolutely necessary. You need to be comfortable, because you will not be able to meditate successfully, if you are uncomfortable and have to keep moving about.

Having got settled, closed your eyes, and slowed your breathing right down, you need something to meditate about. You can select an idea, either spiritual or more mundane, and consider every aspect of it; meditate on it in other words. For many people, however, meditation means repeating a sound, or word, or phrase – a mantra– over and over to themselves; virtually any peaceful, sooth-ing sound, word, or phrase will do. You can do this out loud, or say it silently to yourself. Some people like to chant as a way of meditating, others like to concentrate on some form of image in the mind; another way is to concentrate on your breathing and keep counting the breaths you take. All these ways aim to concentrate the mind and stop it hopping about from thought to thought, as it so often does. If you find your thoughts wandering, you just gently bring your mind back to whatever it is supposed to be doing, without getting upset.

If you are going to try repeating a word over and over again in your mind, you might try words such as 'relax', or 'peace', or 'love'. If you want to try repeating a phrase, you could try something like 'relax, be still', saying 'relax' to yourself as you breathe in and 'be still' as you breathe out; or you could try 'relax, there's no real danger', as a very positive and practical message. Some people like to use a directly religious phrase, such as 'God is love', or 'God is peace'. If you would like to try using an image, you might imagine a lighted candle, or some other form of light. Here you are getting back more directly to a form of visualisation. Whatever you decide to say or do, try to feel relaxed and at ease all the time; to feel that you really can relax, because there is no real danger. Like the visualisation, try to do it with total dedication and sincerity, believing in what you are doing. If you practise regularly in this way, your confidence and belief in what you are doing will grow and then you will really start to get benefits from what you are doing.

The first and most obvious benefit of meditation is that, for a time, you become physically and mentally relaxed and you cease to stress yourself and you cease sending stress messages to your body – your mind cannot send stress messages to your body, if it is concentrating on something else. However strange the idea of meditating may seem to you at first, therefore, it is clearly a good and useful thing to do and the more you practise it, the more benefit you will get from it. It starts to make you more consciously aware of the stress in your life and of the fact that you can do something about getting rid of that stress.

Many people also find, however, that meditation, conscientiously practised, starts to bring them added benefits after a time. It can start to bring a greater sense of tranquillity into every phase of your life; a realisation that all the rush and frantic activity of modern life is not always necessary. It can help to get life into much better perspective and help you to sort out what is and what is not important in life. It can also bring space and stillness into your life and time for a greater awareness of the beauty and mystery of life and of our part in the pattern of Creation. It can help you towards a sense of the peace which passeth all understanding and be a spiritual, as well as a mental and physical de-stresssing.

As I said, you can also practise meditation in a group. In group meditation, everybody gets relaxed, with eyes closed, then one person talks to the group, perhaps taking them in their imaginations on a walk through a beautiful, peaceful countryside or garden, maybe with a crystal clear lake, where they can drink the water, or bathe in the water, if they wish; or maybe taking them to some special place, to which they can always return, whenever they feel in need of peace. Sometimes background music is played, either throughout the spoken part, or afterwards, whilst everyone is still for a few minutes. There are many meditation tapes on the market of this type, which can be helpful, if you wish to practise meditation of this type on your own at home.

There is another technique you can use, which is perhaps not strictly meditation in the true sense of the word, since it aims to still the mind completely, rather than concentrate it on something. This is to sit outside in the garden, or anywhere in the open air, with your eyes closed, and then just be aware of all the sounds and feelings, without attempting to identify or analyse them. Hear the car going up the road, but do not tell yourself, ah yes, that's a car; just hear the noise. Hear the birds singing, feel the breeze in your face, hear the rustle of the trees, feel the chair beneath you, feel the ground under your feet. Just be aware of all these things. It is difficult, of course, to sit there and stop yourself thinking of anything; we spend virtually all our time thinking. You may end up saying to yourself, "I must think of nothing, I must think of nothing", which is not quite the idea. If you practise it, it does become a little easier, though you may never achieve real stillness for more than brief moments, because you can find yourself thinking about the stillness and that thought breaks the stillness. Another way is to sit and look at something such as a flower, again without thinking about it, what colour is it for instance, what shape, what size it is, or even that it is a flower. None of these 'unthinking' methods is easy and the mantra type of meditation is probably the most rewarding way for the majority.

The best thing to do is to experiment and find the way of meditating which suits you best, and then practise it regularly. As with visualisation, it is better to do it well for ten minutes, rather than badly for twenty minutes; quality is important, so get the quality right and then extend the quantity; it does have a cumulative effect. Of the two therapies, visualisation and meditation, I think visualisation is the one on which you should initially spend more time, because it involves you directly and positively in your own healing and helps to strengthen your determination to fight and beat your cancer. Try to fit in at least one session of meditation every day, however, because it does start to bring a greater sense of peace into your life, if you do it conscientiously. It may sound paradoxical to talk of fighting your cancer and reaching a sense of peace in almost the same breath, but the two things are not mutually exclusive. You must fight, if you are to beat your cancer. The sense of peace, as you start to achieve it, will help to relieve the stress you have been under, which made it necessary for you to fight.

To practise both visualisation and meditation every day is time consuming, but if you have cancer, or any other serious illness, you must now spend much more time on yourself, if you really wish to get better. Reinforce the sessions of visualisation and meditation by reminding yourself constantly, as often as you can, to relax and be relaxed. There are some dangers in life that it is best to avoid, but most of the dangers we perceive are purely within our minds and we merely think they are dangers. Keep telling yourself, "relax, there is no real danger". This leads on to some other messages you should start sending to your body.

12

Getting the Messages Right

Too much stress in your life means that you are continually sending the wrong messages to your body; wrong in the sense that the final end result for you is physical illness. The messages need to be changed into good, healing messages and this you will automatically start to do to some degree as you come to see that most of your dinosaurs are indeed only paper dinosaurs and so not really dangerous at all; with a bit of practice, you can learn to deal with them quite easily and so make your life less stressful.

All of us, however, so often send stress messages to our bodies unconsciously, without really thinking about what we are doing, because it has become such a habit to do it. To break this habit more quickly, and therefore to speed up the healing process, it is very helpful consciously to start sending relaxing and healing messages to the body, so that it becomes a habit to send useful, rather than harmful messages. Again, at first, it may seem an odd or childish thing to do. In fact, it is another important way of directly and positively involving yourself in your own healing; another way of strengthening your determination to fight your cancer, and another way of increasing your confidence and belief that you can fight it successfully.

The most important of the right messages are:
'I can relax and let go of my fear; there is no real danger, if

81

I stop doing what my parents told me to do; I am a grown up adult and I am free to do things in my own way now';

'I can relax and let go of my fear; there is no real danger, if I tell the other difficult people in my life to go jump in the lake; I am quite free to do this; they are only paper dinosaurs and, although they may huff and puff a bit at first, they cannot eat me up';

'I can relax and let go of my fear; there is no real danger, if I stop spending all my time looking after others and start spending a bit of time looking after myself for a change; I do not have to please everyone else in life and try to buy their love; I am free to be my own person';

'I can relax and let go of my fear; there is no real danger, if I express my emotions openly in future, rather than suppressing them; I no longer need to go on accepting stress in my life without protest; I am free to control my own life';

'I can relax and let go of my fear; there is no real danger, because my body knows how to heal itself, it wants to heal itself, and it will heal itself, if I learn to get the stress out of my life; I do not have to rely on fate or the whim of God; I have been given the power to heal myself and I am free to heal myself';

Above all, the right message is: 'I can relax and let go of my fear; I am not going to die, because I have too much to enjoy and too much to live for'. Use the cancer itself to strengthen your determination to live and enjoy your life to the full from now on. It has given you a second chance to do this; do not waste that chance.

Make a list of good messages, which apply particularly to you; keep reminding yourself of these messages and keep sending them to your body, every day. Look at yourself in the mirror and say the messages out loud to yourself. At first, understandably, you may not have one hundred percent faith in the messages. Never mind, keep on sending them; you are shutting out the wrong messages. Gradually you will start to build up real confidence and faith in the right messages; you will make them work for you and heal you, just as the wrong messages worked for you and made you ill. It is confidence in your ability to heal yourself that you need to go on and on building up, day after day. You can succeed in healing yourself.

13

Mind over Matter

It may appear that what I have been saying throughout this section on mental stress is that everything is really just a question of mind over matter. Essentially it is, for mind can make us ill and mind can make us well. It is best to be careful, however, when talking about things being mind over matter. All of us have three 'persons' in us, parent, child and adult. My parent is the part of me which absorbed all those do's and don'ts I was taught by my actual parents, and by the other teachers, religious and non-religious, in my life, and which now believes it must itself go on teaching them. My child obeys, or disobeys, more meekly, or less meekly. My adult tries to keep the peace and get on with life, more or less successfully.

If, therefore, my parent insists that it is only mind over matter and would my child kindly get on and do as it is told, my child may start its task, but then take fright, because it considers the task to be an awesome one, and insist that it cannot do it. Alternatively, it may start the task, get bored, because it decides it would be more fun to go out and play, and give up. Child can 'prove' that matter is stronger than mind.

It is very important, therefore, to get the adult in us more in control of our lives. The best way to accomplish this is to start to listen and see who is actually doing the talking, when you speak; is it your parent, your child, or your adult? Sometimes you can catch your parent or your child carrying on in rare old fashion, maybe your parent insisting that your child do its duty and do something it does not want to do, or maybe your child trying to get out of doing its duty and not have to do something it does not want to do. You have to step back and observe what is going on – and it is your adult which can do this of course. Your adult may sometimes decide that it is your adult talking – bully for you! It is interesting to do this with other people as well, when they are talking to you, to see whether it is their parent, or their child, or their adult doing the talking to you. It helps you to realise what the conversation is really about and therefore what you need to do about it. It also helps you to keep a better eye on yourself.

Our moral parent can be a pain sometimes. It is our moral parent who insists to our child that it is our duty to subordinate our own desires and needs to those of our husband, or our wife, or our children, or our parents, or sometimes of seemingly just about everybody else in the world. An aggressive parent in a husband can frighten the wife's child into looking after him, to the exclusion of herself. Wives have sometimes been known to have an aggressive parent in them too. It is precisely when our needs are never met, that we lose a sense of our own worth, and maybe a sense of purpose in life. The irony about an aggressive parent is that it is the cover for an uneasy and frightened child in that same person. People whose adult is largely in control are usually pretty much at ease with themselves and do not have a parental need to be over-aggressive, or over-moralistic; nor do they have a childish need to be over-submissive. Both parent and child in us can, of course, be aggressive, and both can be submissive. Adult keeps the balance, not cold bloodedly, but with compassion, understanding the frailties of both parent and child.

Whenever you feel anxiety and stress, therefore, it will normally be your parent putting pressure on your child to do things your child does not really want to do, for one reason or another, or your child responding to pressure from outside. In pressure situations, whilst child may feel anxiety, adult looks at the situation, decides what can be done, and does it. If adult makes a mistake on the way, as all human beings do from time to time, adult treats this as an interesting learning experience, not an occasion for parent to chastise naughty, careless child. To be adult, is to be free; free of the pressure and stress brought on by the parent/child strife in ourselves, and between ourselves and others – free of the stress which is almost certainly at the root of our illness.

All the various parent and child lessons are, of course, taught to us largely unwittingly by our real parents and it might just be salutary to ask ourselves what lessons we are now unwittingly teaching our own children. It is in your adult role that you can recognise the anger, fear and sorrow which have built up over the years, and as adult that you can recognise that you must direct these emotions in the right direction, express them and let them go. The anger you feel against others for the difficult time they give you in life, and the consequent fear and sorrow you feel, can give way to forgiveness, as you learn, in an adult way, to deal with your difficult people more effectively and see that you no longer need to fear them. They are paper dinosaurs, more to be pitied than feared, for they too were taught the wrong lessons in childhood.

I am asked on occasion whether holistic healing might not make too many demands on patients and might not therefore make them feel guilty, if they cannot succeed in healing themselves. The guilt feelings are the child at work again, feeling guilty because it is disobeying parent healer by not getting better. If you start to feel guilty like this, your healer has not established an adult-to-adult relationship with you and healing does not work well in such circumstances.

The other point which is sometimes raised is that, if patients start to feel and express anger against members of their own family, and then still die, their life and death will have been made more miserable for no purpose. Once again this is a case of poor counselling. If patients do die quickly, clearly they will not have had much time to release anger, but a sensitive healer will be aware of the situation and will help a patient to die in peace despite this. A sensible healer will anyway first discuss with you, on an adult-to-adult basis, whether or not you do wish to fight for your life, and will make sure that you understand what this will entail.

In illness it is easy for us to revert to the child role, demanding love and attention. Some healers give in to these demands and weep with their patients. This is emotional involvement which we should all limit to our own nearest and dearest. If your healer does this, it will not be helpful to either of you. A healer who reacts emotionally with a patient is encouraging that patient to remain in the child role. Patients have to be helped and encouraged to give up the child role and adopt the adult role. It is our adult which can take responsibility for us and for our health. Healers who make a habit of becoming emotionally involved with their patients will anyway burn themselves out sooner or later and cease to be of any help to anyone. Adult healers are compassionate and can understand their patients' feelings, without needing to share them. Adult healers keep their own parent and child under control.

Ultimately, the real lesson which holistic healing should teach you is that you are free to start living a much more purposeful and enjoyable life – and you may start right now. Your adult must therefore learn to give as much scope as it reasonably can to the more delightful, fun-loving, creative side of your child. We need as much fun and laughter in our lives as we can get. Your parent may, of course, try to grumble at all this unseemly behaviour, but a firm hand from adult should put paid to that. We do need to accept that we are three persons, adult, parent and child, for that is what we are. When your adult has your parent and your child on a light but firm rein, however, you will have your emotional life much more in balance and you will be your own person, in control of your life. You will still feel anger, fear and sorrow sometimes and you must make quite sure that you express these emotions – there are plenty of things in this world about which we should feel anger, fear and sorrow, including some of the personal situations which arise in our lives. You should be able to feel your emotions and use them appropriately, and not suppress them. You should be able to deal with them quickly and easily, in an adult way. Since adults see the world as it is and realise that it is not too dangerous, adults have a lot of time to have a lot of fun with their friends. When adult controls mind, adult controls matter, and life goes with a swing.

14

Correcting the Physical Stress Factors

If mental stress is often the most important factor in serious illness, physical and spiritual stress are usually at least contributory factors and they need to be eliminated as far as possible. I will start with the physical factors.

A great deal of the physical stress we suffer does come as the result of our mental stress, of course. Our mind tells our body there is danger about and our body, receiving this message, tenses up so that we are ready to do something about the threat. It can become a habit to hold ourselves tense and a state of slight tension can come to feel much more natural than a state of relaxation. If you eliminate your mental stress, you should in theory eliminate much of your physical stress. In practice, you may not, just because it has become such a habit to be physically uptight. It will help, therefore, to practise physical relaxation directly, so as to help break the pattern of physical tension. There are also other direct physical stress factors and I will look at these as we go along. Even with physical stress factors, your mind is going to have to be involved all the time, because mind tells body what to do; they are interlinked and they always work together.

I have already talked about the need to learn to breathe in a slow, relaxed fashion and about how to learn to do this. It is worth repeating that this is the basis of all physical relaxation. Think of slow, relaxed breathing as a way of giving yourself a free, internal massage. Breathe oxygen into every cell of your body and feel it gently massaging every cell, easing your tensions. Keep massaging the tension out of yourself with your gentle, relaxed breathing.

Breathing leads on to exercise. Many of us lead a very sedentary life these days. We sit, perhaps in hunched up positions, perhaps in unsuitable chairs, for long periods of time. We were meant to be active, outdoor creatures, but we no longer are. The 'good health' point of exercise is not to develop bulging muscles, it is to develop a fit and supple body, which moves freely and easily. One particularly important part of the body, which needs to be as supple as possible, is the spine, because it carries the body's main nervous system and nerves go out from the spine to the various organs of the body. If the vertebrae of the spine become misaligned, nerves can get irritated or trapped. The muscles in that area then try to compensate and ease the pain for you, but can end up tense and cramped; you have developed back trouble. Hanging by your hands from a bar for a few moments a day can sometimes be helpful for minor back troubles, because the weight of the legs stretches the spine and releases pressure on trapped nerves. Swimming can also help, but it would be wise to consult a qualified chiropractor or osteopath if the trouble does not clear up quickly. Cancer patients who develop back pains or other unusual pains should see their doctor or consultant to check for any spread of their cancer.

Obviously, if you have got out of the habit of exercising, take it gently to begin with. Work up to ten minutes of suppleness exercises every morning, aiming to get all the moving parts of the body supple. First thing in the morning, when you have just got up, is a good time. A regular swim, once or twice a week, is first class exercise. Get in some brisk walking, whenever you can. Turn on the radio and dance to the music for a while every day; loosen up and enjoy yourself. Sing along to the music as well. Get some air into your lungs and feel it getting to every cell in your body. If you feel you need a little help

towards getting supple, Alexander and Feldenkrais movement techniques, yoga, T'ai Chi, or gentle aerobics are all
excellent, providing they are well taught by qualified
instructors. Those with arthritis, multiple sclerosis, or
other illnesses affecting the joints, will need to give much
more attention to regaining physical suppleness and will
have to put in a great deal of hard work. Few seem
prepared to do this, though this may be partly because
nobody has convinced them that they can in fact make
considerable improvements by hard work.

It can often help to ease tense muscles, if you first tense
them up even more, before trying to relax them. If you
have a stiff neck, for instance, try to tense up the stiff
muscles more tightly, then release the tension and really
try to feel the muscles relaxing. In a general relaxation
exercise, you can work through your body, starting at the
feet. Tighten up your toes and then relax them; tighten up
your calves and then relax them, and so on right through
your body. Applying the extra tension first allows you to
relax more fully when you release the tension.

A physically relaxed posture is also important. Ideally,
we shall be well balanced, well centred, and we shall walk
through life calmly and with an even step. It will help to
pay conscious attention to posture, so as to ensure that
you do hold yourself in an easy, relaxed manner and that
you can move in an easy, relaxed manner. When you are
standing therefore, make sure that your weight is evenly
balanced and that you do not have all your weight on your
toes, or all your weight on your heels. Your knees should
not be braced back, but should be slightly relaxed. Make
sure that your buttocks are not clenched; lower back
troubles can come from clenched buttocks. Your stomach
should not be pulled in, nor your chest pushed out. Your
arms, shoulders, neck and face should feel relaxed. Your
head should move easily on your neck. Try to imagine that
a piece of string is attached to the top of your head, gently
pulling you up, and that your whole body hangs loosely
and easily from this string. Keep checking to see that

tension does not build up in any part of your body. Once you have regained a measure of suppleness, you can go on to take some more vigorous exercise, in whatever way you enjoy most. Fitness is important, if you wish to feel really healthy, and be really healthy.

Next you have to think how you are going to feed this relaxed, fit and supple body you are aiming to have. Unfortunately, our food has become more and more processed and chemicalised over the years; very little of it is now truly natural food. This adulterated food may not directly kill us; but it can put extra strain on our immune systems by allowing a gradual build up of chemical toxins in the body, which the body's immune system finds increasingly difficult to deal with. The same applies to chemicals used in the home and the environment generally. Just as some of us are more affected by mental stress, some of us will be more affected by the physical stress of the wide range of chemicals used in agriculture, in animal husbandry, in food production, and in the environment. Anyone with any chronic illness should take this into account.

One of the greatest advocates of physical body cleansing, to get rid of these effects, was the late Dr Max Gerson, who taught what came to be known as the Gerson therapy in his clinic in Mexico. Dr Gerson died in 1959, but his work has been carried on by his daughter and granddaughter. Dr Gerson was against orthodox medical treatment for cancer, or for any other serious illness come to that, arguing that illness is caused by this build up of toxins in the body, leading to damage to the liver and other essential organs of the body, with a diet of processed and chemicalised food also leading to a build up of sodium in the body and an increasing deficiency of potassium and iodine. Dr Gerson believed that just two things are necessary to cure illness. These are, to carry out an intensive nutrition programme, flooding the body with easily assimilated nutrients needed to improve healing and metabolism, and to carry out an intensive detoxification of the body to eliminate toxins and waste matter interfering with healing and metabolism.

Dr Gerson paid little or no attention to the possibility of mental or spiritual stress in his patients' lives, believing that, once their liver and other essential organs were restored to health, they would be able to deal themselves with their psychological and spiritual problems. This is at least an admission that these problems do need to be dealt with, though to think that patients will always be able to deal with them themselves, without help, is optimistic in the extreme. Since the Gerson therapy is a very tough and stressful therapy, it might of course be argued that anyone who can stick to the therapy for the length of time necessary is anyway going to be a very determined person to start with.

The main element in the Gerson nutritional programme is juice therapy. Patients are required to drink thirteen eight ounce glasses of selected fruit and vegetable juices a day, one every hour. The fruit and vegetables from which the juices are prepared must be organically grown and the juices must be freshly prepared each hour in special juice presses and drunk right away. The juices used are orange, apple, apple and carrot, grape, grapefruit, and 'green leaf', which is a mixture of vegetable leaves with added sprouted seeds and grains. Very large quantities of organically grown products are therefore needed each week for the juices. Originally, three glasses of juice each day were of calf's liver juice, from calves reared without the use of chemicals, and patients were also give a daily injection of liver extract. The liver injections are still given, but the liver juices have now been discontinued and replaced by extra carrot juices, due to the difficulty of obtaining sufficient suitable liver. Although these liver juices were thought to be important in the beginning, the Gerson Institute say that their results have not suffered since they have been discontinued. In addition to the juices, a variety of different tablets and substances have to be taken during the day at various intervals, including potassium and iodine.

The Gerson diet is a very restricted vegan diet, cutting out meat, fish and dairy products, at least in the beginning. The vegan diet cuts out meat, because our intestinal system is not designed for meat eating and because of the chemicals used in animal rearing. It cuts out dairy products, because they tend to be mucus forming. The Gerson diet is salt free, virtually fat free, and allows very little sugar or other sweetners. A typical Gerson breakfast will be a glass of juice, oatmeal porridge cooked in water, with fruit, followed by rye bread plain or toasted, with a little honey, but no butter or margarine. A typical Gerson lunch or dinner would be a glass of juice, salad, a glass of special vegetable soup, a baked potato and cooked vegetables, followed by fresh or stewed fruit. Extra fruit may be eaten between meals and, after a few weeks, salt free cottage cheese may be added to the salads.

For the detoxification side of the therapy, Gerson patients have to give themselves at least five coffee enemas a day, one every four hours; the coffee must be organically grown and the water must be distilled water, as must any water used for any purpose in the Gerson therapy. To use coffee may seem strange, but it is used because in an enema it is absorbed through the haemorrhoidal and portal veins into the liver, which stimulates the flow of bile, so speeding detoxification of the liver. On top of this, every other day patients must drink two tablespoons of castor oil and, some hours later, give themselves a castor oil enema.

The detoxification process produces reactionary flare ups, as the body starts to re-absorb and eliminate tumours and the toxic products of the years of chemicals and drug residues in the body. The worse the initial state of the patient, the stronger may be the first reactionary flare ups. Flare ups may make the patient feel feverish, nauseous and weak; the patient may suffer intestinal spasms and have pain, and may have severe mood swings, feeling very angry or very depressed, to the point of wishing to give up the therapy. Other old complaints may reappear temporarily and scars and operation and tumour sites may become inflamed and painful. Flare ups are to be taken as a good sign that the therapy is working; they are not a reason for panic and abandoning the therapy. It can be positively dangerous to attempt to alleviate the flare up symptoms with orthodox medical treatment, because this will suppress them and the resulting body toxicity may overwhelm the patient and may even cause death.

If a flare up occurs, patients can help to ease the situation by increasing the frequency of coffee enemas to every two hours, or even more often, continuing them throughout the night as well, so as to speed up detoxification. Flare ups can usually be controlled within one or two days in this way. The first flare up is usually the most violent and, as patients progress, flare ups become less violent and less frequent. Any nausea experienced during flare ups can be eased by drinking large quantities of peppermint tea. A very little honey or raw sugar and a slice of lemon can be added to the tea, if desired.

Coffee enemas can help considerably to ease pain and some patients get a great deal of relief from them. Localised pain can often be eased by wetting three layers of lint with castor oil and placing them on the painful area, covered by a piece of plastic and with a hot water bottle or heat pad on top of the plastic.

Although the Gerson therapy has come to be associated mainly with the treatment of cancer, it is not specific to cancer and the Gerson Institute have found it is equally effective with other chronic illnesses. Cancer patients with other illnesses have found that their other illnesses also clear up with the therapy.

The Gerson therapy has to be carried out by cancer patients for eighteen months to two years and for at least the first six to nine months patients need to give up any form of regular work. Even at the Gerson clinic, where

some help is available, the therapy must clearly be
immensely time consuming and it could become stressful,
tiring and monotonous. Doing it on your own at home, it
must be almost impossible without considerable assis-
tance. This is well brought out by Beata Bishop in her
book 'A Time to Heal', published by New English Library.
She successfully undertook the Gerson therapy to defeat
her cancer and her book makes fascinating reading. Her
book also brings out, however, the lack of any psychological counselling at the Gerson clinic and her need to seek
this elsewhere, as an essential part of her recovery. This
disregard for the mental and spiritual stress factors is, I
believe, a major shortcoming of the Gerson therapy,
which is essentially a very tough physical therapy,
demanding immense courage and dedication, if it is to be
successful. Beata Bishop's book makes very clear that it
can be extremely successful, as does Dr Gerson's own
book, 'A cancer therapy; results of fifty cases', published
by Totality Books. More details of the therapy can be
found in Dr Gerson's book. The Gerson Institute in
California will also provide information and can give
useful contacts in the U.K. Their address is, The Gerson
Institute, P.O. Box 430, Bonita, California 92002, U.S.A.
Their telephone number, dialled from the U.K., is, 010 1
619 267 1150.

Some may feel able to undertake the complete Gerson
therapy, but others will not. Those who do not feel able to
undertake the therapy must, I believe, still consider some
method and degree of bodily detoxification, whether it is
cancer or some other chronic illness they have. Detoxification of the body must help to strengthen the immune
system and therefore help it to defeat the illness.

It is interesting that originally Dr Gerson offered little
hope to any patient who had had chemotherapy, believing that the additional strain chemotherapy inevitably
puts on an already severely toxic body would prevent
healing. Today however, Gerson patients who have had
chemotherapy are put on a less vigorous therapy, in the

belief that this may allow their bodies to detoxify more slowly, so that they may stand a better chance of not being overwhelmed by the toxins released into the body. Patients still take thirteen juices a day, but each juice is four ounces, not eight ounces. Patients take only three coffee enemas a day and do not take the more drastically purging castor oil treatment. They take the same additional tablets as other Gerson patients, but in reduced quantities for some of these. They also take three to four grams of vitamin C a day.

Whilst therefore the Gerson Institute would no doubt claim that the full Gerson therapy should be used whenever possible for cancer patients, the modified treatment for patients who have had chemotherapy does suggest that it might still be useful for any cancer patient, or patient with any chronic illness, even if the healing process were thereby to take longer. Each patient must decide for themselves what they are prepared to undertake, with the proviso perhaps that, if the form of therapy they adopt is not producing the required results, they should be prepared to step up all aspects of the therapy they are using.

An alternative to the Gerson therapy is the rather less restrictive vegan diet suggested by the Bristol Cancer Help Centre, combined with the vitamin and mineral programme they recommend, as a means together of cleansing and building up the body. The Bristol Centre was set up in 1980. It has since become less strict as regards diet, having found that very strict dietary rules were too stressful for some patients, which merely added to their stress problems. The Bristol Centre originally suggested coffee enemas, but later took these out of its programme, relying on the vegan diet for body cleansing. Some vegetable juice may be taken in this way by Bristol patients in the form of carrot juice, if they take the vitamin A or beta carotene which the Bristol Centre recommends. Patients are encouraged to drink fruit and vegetable juices, but no specific quantities are laid down. The

Gerson insistence on such large quantities of juices is because they believe that these provide vitamins and minerals to the sick body in a more easily assimilable form than do vitamin and mineral tablets.

The vegan diet used now at the Bristol Cancer Help Centre is explained in 'The Bristol Recipe Book', by Sadhya Rippon, published by Century; the book also contains many recipes used at the Centre. Patients are encouraged to try the diet and stay on it for at least three months, and longer if they will. It is a salt free, sugar free, low fat diet, with similarities to the Gerson diet, but with a far wider range of 'allowed' foods. Like Gerson, it lays emphasis on organically grown fruits and vegetables. The wider range of foods it allows includes items such as nuts, beans, lentils, whole grains such as brown rice, wheat, barley, oats, rye, maize and buckwheat, and wholemeal pastas.

The Bristol Centre vitamin therapy normally includes quite large doses of vitamins A and C, with smaller doses of other products. Vitamin A is recommended in doses up to 25,000 i.u. per day, or the equivalent in beta carotene or carrot juice. If the palm of the hand starts to turn yellow from large quantities of carrot juice, the amount should be cut back until normal colouring is restored. Vitamin C dosages may start at 2 gms per day, working up to 6 or even 10 gms per day. If there is any sign of diarrhoea as the quantity is increased, the dosage should be reduced until the diarrhoea ceases. Vitamin C in the form of calcium ascorbate may be preferable to ascorbic acid, if ascorbic acid causes acidity, or digestive problems. If you do take large doses of any vitamins, do not stop them suddenly when you do want to stop them. Cut them back gradually over a period of a few weeks, so that your body becomes accustomed more easily to doing without them.

Other vitamins which may be recommended are vitamin E, 100–400 i.u. per day; selenium, 200 mcg per day; zinc orotate, 15 mg per day; evening primrose oil, 500 mg three times daily; and vitamin B, particularly if the patient's energy is low. This may be taken as B complex to include some B12, which is necessary with a vegan diet. In addition, a herbal mixture may be recommended as a detoxifying agent, particularly for those with liver cancer. Those interested in a homoeopathic approach will probably be advised to contact the Royal London Homoeopathic Hospital through their G.P.

The range of options open to patients is clearly very wide. The Gerson therapy, for instance, would expect patients to refuse any further orthodox medical treatment for their cancer, arguing that this would merely further damage an already badly damaged body. The Bristol Centre would be prepared to discuss with their patients any form of treatment the patients wished to consider, orthodox or otherwise.

I myself believe that many patients might benefit from the increased and more rapid body detoxification, which coffee enemas, and possibly also castor oil enemas, might provide, if this is combined with an increased intake of organic fruit and vegetable juices. The more ill the patient, the more this course might seem to be indicated, since time is at a premium. Some patients, in any case, will need a greater degree of detoxification than others. The choice of what to do belongs to the patient and not to the healer or the consultant. Anyone undertaking a Gerson type therapy should be quite certain that they understand it thoroughly, however, and that they understand that it can be dangerous to attempt to suppress flare ups, as and when these occur.

It might be possible to use the modified form of Gerson therapy which is now offered to patients who have had chemotherapy, while still keeping up a nine to five job. One difficulty is that flare ups can occur very quickly, without warning. Another is the juices, since these should be prepared freshly and drunk right away. They lose vitamin and mineral content if they are kept for a few hours. You could take them to work in thermos flasks, but this is obviously a poor second best. It is also possible to buy bottles of organically produced vegetable juices, and sometimes also fruit juices, at some health food shops, but this is even less desirable from a goodness point of view in the Gerson therapy. The coffee enemas might be arranged one in the early morning and two in the evening, when you return from work, though late evening enemas may give you disturbed nights, which will make you tired. All in all, it is probably far better to give up thoughts of work for several months, if you are going to take up this form of therapy.

Again, I would emphasise that whatever form of 'physical' therapy you adopt, it must be combined with effective counselling. Mental and spiritual cleansing and de-stressing are as vital as physical cleansing and de-stressing.

On the practical side, if you decide to try the enema and juices route, you may be able to buy an enema kit from your local chemist; if not, a large chemist in your nearest city or large town should be able to get one for you. A kit consists of a container, usually plastic, for the enema liquid, fitted with a handle so that you can hang it up, and a length of tubing, with a tap at one end and a suitable nozzle at the other end. The tap end of the tubing screws into the bottom of the container. If you have trouble getting what you need, the Gerson contacts in the U.K. will be able to help and advise.

For the enemas, you can make up a concentrate, putting 12 dessert spoons of ground coffee – not instant coffee – into one and a half pints of water; this water should be distilled water in preference to tap water which contains undesirable chemicals. Boil the coffee for three minutes, then let it simmer for twenty minutes. Strain off the coffee grounds and make the liquid up to a full one and a half pints again. This will give you enough concentrate for four enemas. For each enema take a cup of the concentrate, which will be about a quarter of the total amount, and dilute this with three cups of water; this will give you about one and a half pints of dilute liquid. Warm this a little until you can comfortably still leave a finger in it, then it is ready for use. Keep the remainder of the concentrate in the fridge. If you want to make larger quantities of concentrate, these can safely be kept in the refrigerator for four or five days. If you just want to make up one enema at a time, use three dessert spoons of coffee to one and a half pints of water and use this without diluting it.

The thought of giving yourself an enema can be a bit off-putting at first, but it is very easy and you will find that you quickly get used to doing it. You are going to get a few splashes of coffee around the place, so the bathroom is the best place to take enemas, with some newspapers or old towels covering old cushions to lie on. Have a rug to keep you warm if it is chilly, and take a book or radio to pass the time. You should lie on your right side, with your knees drawn up as you give yourself the enema. Breathe steadily as the liquid is flowing in, to draw it into you. Dr Gerson believed from his observations that the coffee is fully absorbed in ten to twelve minutes, so try to retain the enema for at least that long, or a little longer, say fifteen minutes.

Coming back to diet, you must decide how much you want to change your eating habits, and again this is your decision. Assuming that you are going to make some fairly large changes, you may find it easier to change over a period of weeks, rather than trying to change completely over night, particularly if you are going to try to get the whole family onto the new diet. If the family insist in sticking to their old ways, you may feel you have to compromise to some degree, but there is quite a lot you can do on your own, without much difficulty, and without compromising too drastically. Breakfast for you, for instance, might be oatmeal porridge made with water, with added fruit, as in the Gerson therapy, or maybe made with soya milk, rather than cow's milk. Alternatively, you might have a small amount of sugar free muesli, with plenty of fruit added. Follow this with wholemeal bread, plain or toasted, with a small amount of butter or margarine, and just a little honey or sugar free and artificial sweetener free marmalade.

For lunch or dinner, whatever anyone else in the family wants, you can start with a large mixed salad – it is good to start a meal with raw food, because it gets the digestive enzymes working better. You can add some fruit and you can also add sprouted seeds; they are full of goodness. Sprouted seeds are easy to produce. Your local health food shop will sell seeds for sprouting and simple sprouting trays. Alternatively, you can use an old jam jar, with a piece of muslin to cover the top. Cover the bottom of the jam jar with seeds, put in a couple of inches of water and let them soak over night. Then drain the water off and leave the jar on a window sill for three or four days for the seeds to sprout. Three times a day, rinse the seeds under the tap, then drain the water off, keeping the jar covered with the piece of muslin to keep the seeds clean. When the seeds have sprouted, keep them in a plastic bag in the salad compartment of the refrigerator. Alfalfa seeds, lentils, mung beans and sunflower seeds are good and easy ones to start with, but all beans, grains and seeds should sprout. Occasionally you can replace your salad with a really thick vegetable soup, using as wide a variety of vegetables as you have available.

The main course at lunch and dinner may be more difficult, if your family insist on keeping to meat and two veg. You yourself should try to keep off red meat, which contains a lot of uric acid. White meat and fish are less objectionable, but for a few months at least, it might be better if you can also cut these out and substitute a vegetarian or vegan dish. Do be prepared to stick out for what you want for yourself; it is your life that is at stake, not your family's lives.

Dessert can easily be fresh or stewed fruit. You can also make sure that you eat more fruit during the day, between main meals, just as you can drink extra fruit and vegetable juices. If you buy dried fruit, try to get sun dried, rather than sulphur dried. This is not always readily available, but health food shops do sometimes have some. If you buy currants, raisins and sultanas, try to get ones coated with vegetable oil, rather than mineral oil. Oil is used to prevent the fruit sticking together and you may sometimes be able to get uncoated fruit. Again, try your health food shop.

Try to keep off processed, packaged, tinned and frozen foods as much as possible and stick to fresh foods. Aim to cut out salt and use herbs and spices instead. Aim to cut out sugar as well. Keep off sweets, chocolate, shop cakes and biscuits and anything made with white flour. Use wholemeal bread yourself; if the rest of the family want to eat white bread, let them. Cut out tea and coffee, which both contain caffeine, and get on to coffee substitutes and herbal teas. A little carob powder added to coffee substitutes can enliven the taste and just a little honey or raw sugar can make herbal teas taste better, if you find them a bit insipid to begin with.

If you do manage to get organically grown vegetables – and I think you should try to do this – scrub the skins clean, don't peel them; the peel contains a lot of goodness. If you bake organically grown potatoes, eat the skin as well. If you cannot get organically grown produce, wash the produce you do get in a basin of water with two tablespoons of malt vinegar in it. This will at least wash the chemical residues off the skins.

When you are cooking vegetables, steam them, rather than boiling them in water. This helps to retain the goodness. You can buy an adjustable steamer to fit most sizes of saucepan from many cook shops. Put only a very little water in the saucepan below the bottom of the steamer.

The most important thing is to enjoy your food and really feel that it is doing you good – whether it is organically grown or not. If you feel that you have got to eat it, because that is what the diet says, and you don't enjoy it, you will not digest it properly and you will not get as much goodness out of it as you should. Your diet should not become just one more stress factor for you. It is going to help you to cleanse your body as thoroughly and as quickly as you can, so do try to stick with the diet and make it an exciting new part of your therapy.

Patients who have had stomach or bowel surgery may have particular problems with their diet and may need to experiment to see what they best tolerate. Eating small amounts at more frequent intervals will almost certainly be helpful. Mashing and liquidising foods may also help.

Obviously, if you work or live in a very polluted atmosphere, it is better to change your job, or move, or do whatever is necessary to get the pollutants out of your life. One very obvious pollutant is smoking, and, if you smoke, it is going to be better for you to stop smoking. If you cannot stop completely at once, cut down gradually over a period. If you normally smoke twenty cigarettes a day, count out eighteen, lock any others away, and make certain you only smoke eighteen that day. After a week of doing this, or after a fortnight, if a week seems too short to you, cut down to sixteen a day, and so on. Don't try to be extra good one day and cut straight down to ten; you will almost certainly end up smoking thirty the next day. Your body has got used to a certain amount of nicotine each day and it needs to be weaned off it slowly.

Through eliminating physical stress, you are aiming to achieve a supple, relaxed, freely breathing, cleansed and well nourished body; a body in which there are no physical tension blockages; a body in which the physical energy flows freely and easily. Different therapies talk about the flow of energy, which distinguishes the living from the dead, in different ways, purely as energy, or maybe as life force, or vital force; in China it is called Chi, and in Japan Ki. This life force may be said to flow through meridians, and sometimes there is talk of the need to balance the force, or the yin and yang, or the male and female in us, or the left and right sides of the brain. The energy of life will flow through us freely and in a balanced way, if we are physically fit, supple and well nourished, if we do express our emotions, rather than suppress them, and if we are spiritually at peace and talk easily with our God.

In the next chapter, I shall be looking at things spiritual.

15

Spiritual Stress and Spiritual Peace

You may know the story of the person reviewing their life with God, who said, 'Father, I saw in my life, when times were good, two sets of footprints and I knew that you walked beside me; but, when times were bad, I saw only one set of footprints. Why, Father, when times were bad, did you desert me?' 'It is true', God replied, 'that when times were good, I walked beside you, but, when times were bad, I carried you'.

Spiritual stress is a form of mental stress, only this time we are worrying about whether God is looking after us, or whether God really exists at all. Maybe you feel that if God really existed, He would not have allowed you to get cancer. Once you understand the causes of cancer, you can absolve God of blame and pray for some help. The prayer should not be, 'please God heal me', however. God might just be inclined to remind you that He has given you the power to heal yourself and would you kindly get on and do something about it. I believe that the prayer, 'Thy will be done', reflects this ability we have to heal ourselves and that it is God's will that we should use this power, and God's will that we should be well and enjoy the Garden of Eden. 'Thy will be done' is not some sort of divine lottery, with God only deigning to heal us if He got out of bed on the right side this morning. If prayer is to help you, perhaps you should pray for courage to fight your illness and for strength to keep on fighting until the illness is beaten. If we wish to give glory to God, we should do all we can, with the powers He has given us, to get the body He has given us into proper shape. We might add to our prayers a thank you to God for giving us the power to heal ourselves.

Prayer can help us towards spiritual peace. Another help towards this peace can come from spiritual healing – healing by laying on of hands. Some people shy away from spiritual healing, perhaps because they confuse it with spiritualism. Spiritualism believes that messages can be received from those who have died through a person who acts as a medium. This may be very helpful to some people, but it is not what I am talking about here. Some spiritualists also work as spiritual healers and this can cause confusion. There is nothing too strange about spiritual healing. A mother stroking the feverish brow of her child, or kissing the child better, is performing a healing act. We can all heal to some degree, though some may have a greater aptitude for it than others. We can all learn to play chopsticks on the piano. Some will go on to play more complicated tunes. Some like to play the piano and some do not.

Spiritual healing reminds me of the old joke about the man who was very devout and prayed for hours on end every day. One day he was not feeling too well when he got out of bed, but he got down on his knees and started to pray anyway. After about five minutes it was no good, he was feeling so unwell that he had to stop. It was then, in the silence, that he heard the quiet voice say, 'thank heavens, now perhaps I can get a word in'.

I believe that spiritual healing is about stillness and awareness. God may not speak to us in words, but maybe He does speak to us through our experiences in life – if we will listen. Perhaps the message in the experience of stillness and awareness is, 'I am with you; does it not feel peaceful and safe, when you cease your worried chatter and realise that I am with you'. For a moment we approach the stillness of the peace which passeth all understanding.

The essence of the still, alert awareness is the knowledge that we are not isolated pieces of the vast jigsaw which is Creation, but that we are all slotted into this whole picture, healers and patients together. Every piece of the jigsaw is necessary to complete the picture, which is incomplete without every piece. We cannot stand on a wooden platform outside, looking in at Creation. We seem to get a sense of this, when we talk about our own world being one ecosystem, with everything being interlinked and depending on everything else. To remove one thing from the ecosystem has results eventually on the whole. The correct functioning of everything depends on the whole system, and the correct functioning of the whole system depends on everything within the system.

It is easy to talk in these terms of wholeness. It is far from easy to 'lose' one's individual identity and sense the wholeness of Creation and then 'become' that whole. This may be the ultimate whole in holistic, but it is an extremely difficult concept for us as individual human beings in the present state of our consciousness. I am an individual to myself and I find it virtually impossible to be anything else. I have to be 'me', if I am going to survive in the world, or so it seems to me. The 'I' keeps getting in the way. So, in spiritual healing, the change from a sense of individuality to a sense of wholeness just has to happen, if it will; sometimes perhaps for a moment it does. We each tend to see ourselves as one separate wave, surrounded by other separate waves. We cannot see ourselves as the one moving ocean.

Most spiritual healers would probably say that they merely act as a channel for healing energy to pass through them to the patient. Some speak of God's energy, some of divine energy, or universal energy. Some do not seek to know what it is, but just accept that some form of energy seems to be involved. It has been shown, by wiring up healer and patient to biofeedback machines, that the brainwave patterns of a healer in a very relaxed state can sometimes transfer to the patient. It might be described as one consciousness affecting the other, or a sort of tuning in, getting both minds on the same wavelength, so that the patient becomes as deeply relaxed as the healer. Science also tells us that human bodies are not the 'solid' forms they appear to be as we go about our every day lives. They are forms of energy, millions upon millions of far from solid atoms, all moving and vibrating. If we block that energy through any form of stress or tension, the energy cannot flow easily. In deep relaxation, the energy may flow and vibrate more freely, just as consciousness may flow more freely between healer and patient. The patient's body then has more stress-free conditions and may start to heal itself. The more the healer's sense of relaxation is transmitted to the patient, the greater probably will be the benefit to the patient.

When our energies are flowing freely, we may also be more in tune with the energies flowing all around us, for all matter in the Universe is made up of atoms of some sort; the whole Universe is a moving, vibrating energy form. Our human consciousness has still not developed to the point where we see things this way, but maybe this Universal energy, or divine energy, or God's energy, call it what you will, may also flow more freely through healer and patient, when both are truly relaxed. The more we become conscious of this possibility and the more we allow it to happen, the more perhaps we shall be healed. We become our own channel for our own healing. As our human consciousness develops further and we become more aware of the extent of consciousness and energy, we may start to see through the glass less darkly.

Ancient wisdom speaks of the body having seven main centres of energy – the seven chakras – ranging from the crown of the head to the base of the spine, these chakras being linked to the various glands of the body and reflecting different colours. Many healers use these energy centres in healing; some use colour; some talk in terms of auras around the body and of etheric bodies; some healers use touch more than others. The patient does not really

need to be concerned with the beliefs of the healer to
benefit from spiritual healing; if it works, it works.

Most spiritual healers would say that you do not have to
believe in spiritual healing for it to help you. This can be
true, though it is very doubtful if it is worth going to a
spiritual healer if you positively believe that it is not
going to help you. Conversely therefore, it may help you
more if you positively believe that it is going to help you.
The most important thing is to find a spiritual healer with
whom you feel comfortable. No one healer is for all
patients.

Many patients say that they get a sense of peace during
spiritual healing, though this may not always happen the
first time, when they are not quite certain what, if
anything, is supposed to be happening to them. If they get
nothing more than peace from it, that can still be helpful,
whether or not they give it any religious significance.
Perhaps they can take that sense of peace out into their
lives with them and remember it and practise it. It will
help the physical healing.

What about miracle cures? I have said that we have
more control over our bodies potentially than we ever
allow ourselves to believe. Fakirs, who let themselves be
buried for twenty-four hours and then come up smiling,
have learned to slow their bodily systems right down, as
animals do in hibernation. Fakirs who push needles
through their cheeks, without any sign of blood, are
telling the blood not to flow, with an utter conviction that
they can control the flow of blood – and they do. We can
achieve a very great deal of conscious control over our
bodies; our bodies do what we tell them to do, including
heal themselves, if we tell them what to do with conviction and really believe that they can and will do it. It may
take time.

I read some time ago of an Irish healer who was
apparently the seventh son of a seventh son, and who
claimed to have effected many miracle cures, and to have a
stack of newspaper cuttings to prove it. He said that

miracle cures did not always take place and that he did not know how they happened, when they did happen. If I believe with a deep conviction that a seventh son of a seventh son can definitely perform a miracle of healing on me and go to him fully expecting to be healed, and if, at the very moment I am with him, he also has an absolute certainty that he is going to heal me, then perhaps the miracle will happen. Maybe as his consciousness and my consciousness 'meet', there is for a moment a completely stress-free moment of stillness, in which there is no blockage of energy, physical, mental or spiritual, in either person, and in which we both 'know' with absolute certainty that nothing can prevent me being cured, and so I am cured; the miracle takes place. For the seventh son of a seventh son, we might perhaps substitute any particular spiritual place where miracles are alleged to have happened, or any other person or event associated with such happenings. Miracles are few and far between. Perhaps it is that we do not have the faith which Christ had and we do not inspire the faith which Christ inspired. Whether the miracle cure will last a life time may sometimes be open to doubt. If, after a time, the stress in my life returns and the faith weakens, I might just get a relapse. It is in stories that the prince and princess marry and live happily ever after. In real life, as the years go by, they may start to quarrel and end up in the divorce courts.

Instant miracle cures are quite possible in theory. In practice, for the majority of us, they are not going to happen. Inadvertently we have put in a lot of hard work over the years into making ourselves ill, stressing ourselves, day in and day out. Now consciously, we are going to have to put in a lot more hard work, day in and day out, if we are going to heal ourselves. If we do put in this hard work, day in and day out, we shall heal ourselves. That is the true and lasting miracle – and it is freely available to all of us.

It would save a lot of time, of course, if spiritual healing could regularly produce miracle cures. It doesn't. Occasionally, you may meet a spiritual healer who insists upon telling you about how they witnessed a cancerous lump disappear before their eyes. Such healers should be requested to perform an instant miracle cure on you and told politely that, if they cannot put up, they should shut up.

Our longing for a miracle cure may reflect our fear that we may die. Our fear that we may die may be our fear that God has deserted us and will let us die; our child expects our Father to look after us. It is quite possible to have an adult relationship with God, starting with the under-standing that we can heal ourselves and do not have to rely on God to wave a magic wand over us. Our more adult view of life may help us to extend our consciousness and our understanding of the Creation in which we exist. What today tends to be viewed as paranormal, may well tomorrow become normal. The ways in which we commu-nicate with each other today, and regard as quite normal, might well have been regarded by primitive man, if he had been able to think about it, as very paranormal. Where originally we lived purely by instinct, now we are conscious, and we are aware that we are conscious. Our consciousness has grown over the centuries and we undoubtedly have the ability to extend it further. It should help us to heal ourselves, to reach a more holistic way of living, and to view the Universe in a more holistic way.

Adult understands that, although our consciousness has developed a great deal since the early days, it still has a long way to go and we had better keep our feet firmly on the ground, which is where they belong. If the parent/child conflicts, which exist to a greater or lesser extent in all of us, still prevent us from living in harmony with ourselves and with others, and lead us to making a mess of the garden in which we live, that is our sad loss and it can create a hell for us. As the mess we have made of our garden forces us to face up to what we are doing to it and to ourselves, and forces us to face up to ourselves and the strife we create, this may help our consciousness to develop further. We may begin to see mankind and the garden and the Universe within God, as the whole undivided Creation they are; and that will be our gain and our heaven.

What happens after death, we do not know; it will be interesting to find out. Meantime, through adult, we can learn to heal ourselves and we can learn to heal our garden. That gives us plenty to get on with for the moment.

Some prefer to believe that there is no spiritual side to life; I prefer to believe that there is. I believe that the spiritual message is that we are within the wholeness of Creation and that we cannot fall out of Creation. If we keep adult in control, we keep the potential for evil within ourselves in control, and we walk in the way we are meant to. Then we know we are within this whole Creation and we need have no fear. We can relax, there is no danger.

16

Creativity – Enjoying Life

As you learn to deal more easily with your difficulties and build up your self-esteem, life will begin to be that bit more exciting and worthwhile. The more purpose you find in life, the more you are saying to your body, life is worth living, I do not want to die. It is the most important message you can send to your body. All illness should teach us more about ourselves. Life-threatening illness should teach us what is really important in our lives and what has relatively little value. Some cancer patients will say that they are glad they had cancer, because it showed them the true priorities in life. Cancer can offer a second chance in life. These people were able to use their cancer as an opportunity to achieve a more fulfilling, worthwhile and creative life.

Some patients set themselves targets, as a way of keeping their cancer at bay – 'I can't die for the next six months, because my daughter is getting married in six months' – or whatever the reason may be. This may be very helpful in keeping you going for a while, because it gives purpose to your life. In this sense therefore, it must come under the heading of being 'a good thing'. In another sense, however, it may sadly be the same as the consultant telling you that you have only got six months to live. If you accept that message and send it to your body, your body will probably obey it. It is because your body has obeyed all the danger and stress messages you have

114

sent it over the years that you have cancer. Understand that and you will understand that the last message you should send to your body is that, effectively, you are happy to die in six months. The message that you have to send to your body, and the purpose that you have to have now, is that you are going to die of old age, rather than of your illness. Y our life has to become so full of purpose that you find it quite unacceptable to die of anything but old age, because now you have got so much to do in the meantime. Send that message to your body and you will be far more likely to survive.

Start therefore to create a new and more exciting life for yourself; fill your life with creativity and fill your life with enjoyment and laughter. Real uninhibited laughter is a great healer; you cannot be stressed when you are laughing heartily. Remember that it releases healing chemicals into the body. Concentrate on living in the present, without worrying too much about the past or the future, and live and do everything with enjoyment, with dedication, and with enthusiasm. Find out what you really want to do to fulfill yourself, to use your talents and to develop your talents to the greatest possible extent. For some, this might mean turning in the boring old office job and going off to play in a jazz band at half the salary. It might mean finding a happier relationship, or splurging the savings on a trip round the world and hang the consequences afterwards. For others it may mean more modest projects; joining the local dramatic society, because you always had a hankering to do so, or joining evening classes to learn how to paint, how to do flower arranging, or how to lay bricks. Anything you have always wanted to do, but never have, anything which you think you would like to do and might enjoy doing; anything which, because it is creative in the broadest sense of the word, gives more purpose to your life – something really for yourself, to enhance your life. Start putting aside time for yourself, when you can do what you want to do; maybe an hour a day; maybe half a

day every week. Don't wait to enjoy yourself; start doing
what you want to do now. Life becomes worth living,
when it is full of enjoyment.

Don't be afraid to discuss your life and your life style
with your spouse. Do not go on assuming that your
spouse expects you to go on with the same old routine,
because it is your duty to do so and because it is your duty
to be a good provider for your family. Your spouse is
going to benefit more from having you alive and happy,
than from having you miserable and dead, even if you are
all a bit less well off financially. You do not have to please
everyone else in life either; you do not need everyone
else's love; you will not get satisfactory relationships that
way. Do what you want to do to fulfill yourself and you
will attract to you those of like mind and disposition, with
whom you really can have meaningful and enjoyable
relationships.

Start to look around you a bit more as well and become
more aware of things around you; give yourself time to
stand and stare. Get out into the country, or the local park,
or your own back garden, and become aware of the life in
everything around you. See once again the shape and
colour of flowers and trees; feel them; smell them. Watch
and listen to the birds. Be aware of the sun and the wind
and the rain. Look up at the stars and see the immensity of
the Universe. You are part of it, privileged to see it and
live in it; be aware that it is full of the same life that is
within you. Creation is all around you and its wonders
cost us nothing; they are free for all of us to see and enjoy.

Mythology in many languages and cultures tells of the
hero going on a long journey, of a fight against great
perils, of re-birth and return. The shaman had to make
this journey, so that he might become the tribal healer. He
would recount the story to the assembled tribe, who
would join in, entranced, with dancing and singing and
drumming. By the end, the whole tribe was healed.
Versions of the story appear in pantomime and here too
the audience may join in and become spell-bound, hiss-

ing and clapping, singing and stamping. If the tale is well told, the audience will go away at the end happy and 'healed'.

Holistic healers who are worth their salt will have made their own journey; they will have learned to accept life and themselves and they will know that life is a continuing journey of growth and development. Otherwise, they will be of little help to their patients.

As you are helped to make your own journey and overcome the perils on the way, you will come to the 're-birth' of an understanding and acceptance of yourself, and to the realisation that you do not have to remain trapped in the past. You are free to be yourself and enjoy life and Creation. Add to Creation through your own individuality and your own creativity. Help to sing the continuing song of life.

17

Cancer in Children

Much of what I have written about cancer may not seem to apply to children, since they have not had such a long period of time in which to suppress their emotions. A more obvious possible cause of their cancer can lie in the chemical revolution of the past fifty or so years. The parents of children today were subjected to the increasing flood of chemicals introduced into the food chain and into the environment over the past decades. They were also living in an increasingly fast moving and more stressful world. It is not surprising that some of the children of some of these parents should develop illnesses such as cancer. Children do not have such strong immune systems as adults. Children are also in a period of rapid growth, with their body cells renewing themselves at a faster rate. There is a greater chance of cells developing incorrectly.

In addition, western developed countries appear to have a higher incidence of childhood cancer than less developed countries. These western developed countries themselves had a lower rate of childhood cancer, when they were less developed. In less developed countries children are more exposed to infectious illnesses at an early age, whilst in more developed countries, these infectious illnesses have been eliminated to a great degree by improvements in sanitation and by vaccination and immunisation techniques. In the less developed countries, children may die of the infectious illnesses, but, if they do survive, their early exposure to infectious illnesses seems to give them some protection against contracting cancer later on.

We should also not dismiss totally the possibility of some mental stress in children. I spoke earlier of the need we all have for a great deal of love from our parents in childhood and how lack of sufficient love can stress us. There is a vast range between unconditional love and no love at all and most of us will end up somewhere in the middle of that range. If we end up as children too near to the no love end of the range, we may be in trouble.

There is not necessarily any need for parents to feel guilty on the score of mental stress in their children, however, for not all the children in the same family will be exactly the same; some are born physically stronger than others and similarly some inherit in their genes characteristics, which the others do not inherit. With the best will in the world, it is also almost certain that different children in a family will be treated at least slightly differently. The first child in the family will, for instance, be treated differently from later children, because parents will have more experience to draw upon with their later children. The first child may, of course, have rather too much responsibility put upon it too early in its life, if it is expected to take too large a role in the upbringing of the later children. It may also feel neglected, when the parents' attention, rightly in their view, is directed more towards later additions to the family. If any child in the family is favoured, the others may feel neglected and less loved. What is important in the end is not so much what the parents perceive the situation to be, as what the child perceives the situation to be; that is the reality for the child. If a child is a little more nervous and withdrawn, it may have the impression that it is not receiving as much love and attention as its brothers and sisters, whatever the actual situation may be.

The holistic approach to a child with cancer will obviously depend to some degree on the age of the child and on how much it can understand. Children do have the great advantage of having vivid imaginations and this can be of great use in their healing. Children will also often be aware of just how ill they are. They may take easily to the idea that they can use their imagination to help to make themselves better. Visualisation comes easily to children and can be used in story telling, with the children being encouraged to join in. Relaxed breathing and relaxation come more easily to children than to grown ups. Many children will also take easily to spiritual healing; again it can be combined with story telling, perhaps of a trip to a magic place. Art therapy can also be helpful, since again this uses the child's imagination. Improved diet and extra vitamins and minerals can obviously be introduced for the child. If the child is not too young, it can be put on a modified Gerson therapy of extra organic fruit and vegetable juices, with coffee enemas to detoxify the body. A very young child can be given the organic juices, without the enemas. If a baby is being breast fed, the mother should go on a Gerson type detoxification programme herself.

The parents need to be involved with whatever is being done for the child and they need to understand what may lie behind the child's illness, even if, at first, this is painful for them and even if, rightly or wrongly, they feel some element of guilt. Unless there has been deliberate stress placed upon the child, it may be largely the luck of the draw that one child in the family contracts cancer, whilst the others do not. The whole family must be taught to pull together as a team, however, to help the child who is ill, and they must understand the therapy to be practised.

18

Those Most Likely to Survive

Many cancer patients, including some who are taught holistic ways, do fine for a time, even for a period of years, but then fall ill again with secondary cancer. Maybe this has happened to you. It can be shattering and cause deep despair, particularly if you thought that you had learned the lessons of your cancer and had made what you thought were the necessary changes in your life. You may ask yourself what more you could have done. Maybe you were not well enough taught how to get rid of your stress. Maybe you were initially well taught, but gradually ceased to pay enough attention to yourself, as you started to get better, and slowly slipped back into your old stressful ways.

Almost certainly the patients who get secondary cancer do so because they do not fully face up to the difficulties in their lives and deal with them adequately; they do not sufficiently get rid of the accumulated backlog of suppressed emotions, which was the real, original cause of their illness. The danger starts when you have begun to make changes in your life and find that being assertive really works; it does make the difficult people far easier to handle and life becomes much less stressful and more enjoyable. You feel that you are getting to be in control of your life for the first time. You are no longer a puppet on strings, dancing to other people's tunes. The danger is that you now believe that you have solved everything and that being assertive in public is all you need to do and that you can forget about any past stress. It can be a bad mistake; you just have not got enough stress out of your life.

Subconsciously, you may possibly also feel relief at finding an excuse not to express any anger against your nearest and dearest, even in private, because it does feel wrong to do so. It is also easy to express a bit of token anger for a time and then kid yourself that you have got rid of enough for you to say that you forgive those who have made such difficulties for you in your life. It makes you feel good and it makes you feel as if you have done your duty by forgiving them. Yet again, it may be easy to fool your conscious mind; it is not easy to fool your subconscious mind. If you only shake a little straw off your back, it is only going to be necessary for you to put a little bit more back on again for your back to break again. At this stage, because you have not sufficiently got rid of your backlog of emotions, you are very vulnerable to any additional stress. You may have to go on thumping your pillow. It took years to build up the straw on your back; you are not necessarily going to get rid of it in a couple of weeks. Many cancer patients get rid of a certain amount of stress, but then let it build up again. It is the subconscious stress, or the stress that you are not prepared to acknowledge, which can be so dangerous. Cancer patients, who become helpers in the local cancer support group they attend, sometimes develop secondary cancer, because they take on too much, too quickly. As soon as they begin to feel better after their hospital treatment, they feel they should start to help others, who are now going through the traumatic experiences they themselves had to live through. It is a very worthy motive, but it is easy to slip back into the old stressful habit, which probably they had before, of spending too much time on others and too little time on themselves.

The first symptoms of the renewed build up of suppressed emotion may show up as breathing difficulties and make you worried that the cancer has spread to your lungs. They may show up as aches and pains, which move around and seem to be in the bones; you worry that the cancer has spread to your bones. These may be just symbolic warning signs to you from your body that you are finding it difficult to breathe emotionally, or that life is becoming a pain. Get yourself checked out, without fail, to see whether or not the cancer has spread. Whether it has or not, you go back to thumping your pillow and you go back to spending a lot more time de-stressing and healing yourself, than clearly you recently have been doing. Most patients with cancer probably live with a fear of developing secondary cancer. Understand the stress behind your cancer, physical, mental and spiritual, make sure that you get rid of past stress, and that you cope adequately with future stress, and you will be highly unlikely to get secondary cancer.

Those patients who decide to fight for their lives will stand a better chance of survival. If they are taught to understand the causes of their cancer and taught how to fight, they will stand an even better chance. The same applies to you. The more advanced the state of your illness, the harder you are going to have to fight in the beginning; time is not on your side. Your healer will have to make you angry and aggressive, even if this makes you angry with your healer. It may have to be a case of your healer having to tell you to stop feeling so sorry for yourself and get up off your backside and start doing something about your illness. You need to become extra-aggressive for as long as it takes. If you are not eating much, because eating makes you sick, or because you are afraid it will make you sick, you have to be persuaded to make yourself eat, even if it does make you sick. You have to go on forcing your body to accept food, until your body does accept food. You have to keep your strength up. You also have to keep yourself moving and active, even if you are physically weak. To give up and submit to not taking food and exercise is to continue the old accepting, submissive ways and to continue to send the old accepting and submissive messages to the body. The body will obey. As long as you wish to survive, you must keep fighting.

Of course, you may decide at some time that the struggle is too much. That is your choice and you have the right to make whatever choice you wish; your healer's wishes do not enter into the matter. If your healer has developed the necessary adult relationship with you, you should both be able to discuss your decision in an adult manner. You can then be helped to die as peacefully as possible, hopefully making peace with your friends, with your enemies, with yourself, and with God.

There are some cancer patients who prefer to deny that they are, or have been, seriously ill, though, if you are reading this book, you are probably not one of them. Some of these patients appear to cope in this fashion. If they truly convince themselves that they have not got cancer, and never have doubts on the subject, they may get away with it. Clearly, however, the method has its dangers. Some form of stress has caused their cancer and denying that they have cancer does not necessarily eliminate that form of stress from their lives. If it continues to stress them, sooner or later they may get an upsurge of their illness. Any additional new stress, which comes into their lives, may hasten the process.

Those who resign themselves to their illness will clearly not do so well, but they also would presumably not be reading this book. They do not believe that they have any power to tell their bodies to do anything, despite the fact that their illness proves just how well their bodies have obeyed the messages they sent it. By resigning themselves to their illness, they continue to send these old danger and stress messages. Their inability to believe that they might recover will prevent them from recovering. Effectively, they are telling themselves to die. Our powerful mind can even over-ride our most powerful instinct, our instinct to survive.

Most patients will see the need to make changes in their lives, if the cause of their cancer is made clear to them, and most can quickly be started off in the right direction, if they are properly taught. We are all different, so we shall all progress at different rates. I hope that, by now, you will appreciate the need for changes in the ways you handle your life. Occasionally a patient comes along, however, who seems to find extreme difficulty in facing up to the need for change – and you may just be one of those patients. If so, read on, because it needs saying that such patients were, in their childhood, well and truly brain washed by their parents. Although their lives are now stressful and unhappy, because they are unable to get the love they need, they seem to feel that they cannot change, because, if they changed so that they might get more love and improve their lives, this would somehow mean that they would cease to be true to themselves and to the person they are. They are damned if they do and they are damned if they don't.

To others, this attitude can seem both stupid and cussed, for logic no longer enters into the subject. This unwillingness to change is a measure of the extent to which these patients have been brainwashed by their parents. They have been brought up to be the people they are and taught that this is how they must be, and this is how they must remain. It is their unwillingness to disobey these commands, even though this may kill them, which prompts the term brainwashed. Parents may well do these things inadvertently and they may inadvertently cause their children to get cancer in later life, so the term brainwashed may sound harsh. If it helps to arouse anger in the patient and helps to break the spell of unquestioning obedience to parental commands, then the term is justified. To accept that you may not change your ways and must die because of what your parents taught you in childhood is to continue to act the child to the point of absurdity; it is to reject yourself and your own humanity. If you wish to live, you must find yourself and be yourself. If God reviews our lives with us when we die, I doubt if He will ask us why we did not strive to be as others wanted us. He might well ask why we did not strive to be ourselves.

We need to understand that our minds produce physical changes in our bodies. Our minds are powerful enough to make us ill, and they are powerful enough to make us better. Our bodies have tremendous recuperative, self-healing powers, as even orthodox medical practitioners will be prepared to admit. If we learn to harness the powers of our minds to the self-healing powers of our bodies, we shall achieve seeming miracles. Often we just do not allow ourselves to believe that we might achieve such miracles. Such miracles are well within our powers, if we learn that we must be ourselves and not be the creature of others.

19

So Let's Get the Fear out of Cancer

In this book I have written in the main for cancer patients and their therapists, but it applies to us all, sick and well. We all get stress in our lives and we are never going to succeed in getting the balance of our lives perfectly right all the time. Much of the stress comes because we have been taught in childhood to suppress our emotions to some degree – to sit up, shut up and behave ourselves. We could all profitably spend a few minutes every day venting our emotions in private, because we all tend to pile straw onto our backs. Some of us will need to thump our pillows more violently and more often than others, but we all need to thump our pillows a bit. We also need to make sure that we keep our bodies cleansed and well nourished, and we need to seek some spiritual peace. The physical state of our bodies reflects accurately how we have reacted to stress throughout our lives. The more we get rid of our stress, the healthier we shall be. If we do not do this, orthodox medicine may be able to patch us up for a time, but the continuing stress will probably make us ill again at some time in the future. The danger with orthodox medicine, if that is all that is offered to us, is that it may well leave us still oblivious of the need to deal with the stress in our lives.

Many fear cancer because they do not understand it and because it can be a killer. Many vow that they will beat their cancer, but then do little effectively to achieve this, perhaps because they are not taught what to do. Cancer is a very serious illness, but it is no different to other serious illnesses in that it is most often caused by too much long term mental stress, with physical and spiritual stress merely as contributory factors in some degree or other. Cancer does not come from outer space; it is not caused by something against which you are powerless to act. You can immediately and quite easily start taking steps to de-stress yourself, physically, mentally and spiritually; to get into control of your life, to get into control of your body, and to get into control of your cancer. Certainly it will need dedication and conviction, but there is nothing – apart from yourself – to stop you doing it. Your body knows how to heal itself and wants to heal itself. Give it stress-free conditions and it will do everything it possibly can to heal itself. Gaining faith in your ability to start controlling your cancer will lift an enormous amount of stress from you, because, if you have faith in your ability to do this, you need no longer fear cancer in the same way. Fear of cancer alone can be a tremendous drag on you. Let others call your faith a placebo effect, if they wish, when they see it working. It is not a placebo effect because it is based on the solid fact that our bodies do heal themselves, given the right conditions.

I have written at some length about the mental aspects of stress. If you have cancer, you were almost certainly brought up to believe that you had to do your duty and accept many things in life without real protest; others have effectively controlled your life. Whether you did your duty gladly, or less willingly, you accepted that you had to do it and, eventually, the stress gave you cancer. Your brothers and sisters, if you had any, will have received much the same upbringing as you, but may not have been affected by it to the same degree or in the same way as you. They may have got angry and rebelled against the idea of doing duty, or they may have been more laid back and not felt stressed and not felt that they were under pressure to perform any duty. You probably inherited a slightly different mix of physical and mental characteristics to your brothers and sisters, which made you react to pressure in different ways to them. Maybe you were, or felt you were, treated slightly differently by your parents as well. You drew the short straw in your family and you were therefore the one to develop cancer.

You may have drawn the short straw in your family; that does not mean that you can do nothing about your illness. You have a straightforward choice. You can go on believing that it is imperative that you go on and on obeying what you believe to be the commands of your parents, continually stressing yourself by reacting to others and to life in the ways you learned as a child, even if this eventually kills you, or you can decide that this behaviour is indeed foolish and that you are not prepared to die for this cause. This book has been about what to do, if you decide that you would prefer to live, rather than die.

Do not be discouraged or put off by those who do not believe in holistic therapies, or if your cancer continues to progress at first while you are learning to practise the therapies effectively. You cannot necessarily expect to stop it and reverse it immediately. Set yourself the first more modest target of getting it under control so that, even if it does not get any better, it does not get any worse. Once you have got this much in control, then start to think about actually getting rid of your cancer completely.

Do not be discouraged, even if you now have a recurrence of your cancer for a second or third time. Understand that this shows that you have not yet managed to get enough stress out of your life and that you now have to do this quickly, or you may not get another chance. Seize this chance with both hands now. Don't be discouraged, if you have been told that your cancer is inoperable. Don't even be put off, if your cancer consultants tell you that you have only got months or weeks to live. They are saying to you that there is nothing further that anyone can do for you and that you must go away and die. They are wrong. They have been treating the symptoms of your illness;

you are going to tackle the causes. There may be nothing further they can do for you; there is plenty you can do for yourself. Doing it with real conviction and with real dedication can show you that it does work. Other people make it work and you can make it work. It is no good doing it half-heartedly, or with your fingers crossed behind your back, in case it does not work. It is no good either, hanging around, waiting for someone else to do it for you. You have to do it yourself and it needs all the 'sincerity' you can put into it. Keep doing it with sincerity and belief and you will start to build up the confidence that you can and will succeed.

The true holistic approach is a very simple, down to earth approach. It is important that you keep it that way. There are a confusing variety of so-called alternative therapies on offer in the market place. Health exhibitions, health books and health magazines are full of them, all offering different ways of healing yourself. Some are purely physical therapies, some are therapies aimed at relieving mental stress, some at relieving spiritual stress, some at mixtures of all three. Since many do not clearly explain their limitations, this can make things even more confusing for you. Some therapies can be helpful; some will be less so. The temptation is to assemble together all the ones which seem to offer any sort of help and attempt to undertake them all. You will end up confused, tired, stressed, and quite possibly considerably out of pocket. Rushing from one therapist to another is a sure recipe for disaster.

For most people, it helps to find one good holistic teacher. A good holistic teacher will teach you to walk on your own and will try to see that you get enough help and do not try to walk on your own before you really can. The amount of help you need from your teacher is a point which should be discussed between you. You can also discuss with your teacher whether or not it might be useful for you also to try one or two of the many alternative therapies on offer in the market place and why these might help you. If you cannot find a good holistic teacher, this book can be used as a do-it-yourself manual; it has been written partly with this end in view. This will require rather more self discipline from you, but then all D.I.Y. projects require a certain amount of self-discipline.

I do not wish to knock any of the alternative therapies. You can always find people who have been helped by virtually any therapy; they have faith in it. What the true and simple holistic approach wishes to teach you is to have faith in yourself and in the powers of your body and mind. The greatest therapy of all the therapies on offer is the one that comes free; the ability and desire of our bodies to heal themselves, if we give them relatively stress free conditions, and the power of our minds to send healing and relaxing messages to our bodies, rather than stressing messages, so that our bodies do heal themselves.

Learn to have faith in these abilities which you have, because they are there for you to use, and they work – do not let anyone tell you otherwise. As you develop this faith, everything becomes largely D.I.Y. If you are working on your own and, after proper examination, you really believe that one or two of the alternative therapies could be of real help to you within your healing programme, do by all means incorporate them into your programme. Use them, however, not as permanent crutches, but as a means of helping yourself along for a time, whilst you are learning to walk by yourself. If, when you are better, you feel you would still like to keep on with some form of group exercise or relaxation, which you have been practising, do so, of course. If you feel the need to keep on permanently with an individual therapist, however – and that would include your holistic healer, if you were going to one – you are not being taught, and you are not learning, that you must come to take the prime responsibility for your own health. It is a lesson you must learn.

Success comes from doing a few relatively simple things consistently and well. Let me summarise them.

Remember first of all that your mind does control your

body. Your body does not have a mind of its own, it has your mind and it is your mind that tells your body what to do. Keep reminding yourself of this, because it will keep reminding you not to stress yourself and not to send stress messages to your body. The more you come to realise that you really do have the power to control things, the quicker you will get rid of the fear of cancer. It does not have to control you; you can control it.

Make sure that you understand and acknowledge the stress which you have had over the years and that you understand and acknowledge why you have had it. Make sure that you really do release this stress; thump your pillow as much as you need to. Don't run risks with your life by thinking that you don't need to thump your pillow, however silly it may seem at first. You want to do everything you can to get as much stress out of your life as possible. In private, you can be really aggressive, so as to get this stress out of your system as quickly as possible and prevent it lying around in your subconscious, where it would continue to stress you. Remember, you will not fool your subconscious; if the stress is there, it is there, however well hidden it may be inside you.

Make a habit also of quickly de-stressing yourself at any time in the day that you find yourself getting a bit uptight. If you can, stamp your foot, get angry, and tell yourself out loud that you are not going to accept this stress; then smile and let it go. If you cannot do this, because it is not appropriate at the time, just tense up a bit more, then let the tension go quietly, as you breathe out. Don't be afraid to feel and express your human emotions.

Make sure that you also work hard at being more assertive, so that you do not stress yourself so much in future and so that you are more in control of your life. Take the decisions you want to take; your family and other people do not have to have you look after them all the time. There is no need to go around deliberately being beastly to other people to get what you want, but, equally, there is no need to be afraid that, if you upset other people occasionally, they will cease to love you. You do not have to buy love and you do not have to get everyone else to love you. You must be your own person.

Practise your visualisation regularly every day, because it involves you positively and directly in encouraging your body to heal itself and get back to its original healthy blue-print. Help this along with regular meditation every day, to help you to gain a greater sense of peace and balance into your life, and an awareness of what is important and what is not important to you.

Remember to keep sending the right messages to your body, every day, as often as you can. You are going to control your life now and you are going to enjoy your life now and make it a much more fulfilling and creative life.

Set about cleansing and detoxifying your body and start to make improvements in your diet; this is also an important part of your healing programme. Your body will function better if it is fed the natural foods it was designed to eat, rather than processed and chemicalised foods it was not designed to eat.

Keep practising your relaxed, easy breathing; remember you cannot be physically or mentally uptight if you are breathing in an easy, relaxed manner. Relaxed breathing will help your heart to beat with a steady rhythm and send around your body the steady supply of oxygen and blood it also needs, if it is to function efficiently. Your body does know how to function efficiently, but it cannot and will not do this if you put it under stress and prevent it functioning efficiently.

Look to your spiritual needs as well; we can all do with a greater sense of 'the peace which passeth all understanding'. The one separate wave we now seem to be as an individual being was always in the ocean before we were born and always will be in the ocean when we die, and our wave sinks back into the ocean.

To start with, you will have to do these things I have summarised very consciously and you will have to dedicate time to doing them. Do them with enthusiasm and with the confidence that you really can succeed. Do not pressurise yourself too much, however, if you have a day when you really do feel ill and really do need a bit of a rest. Do still try to do at least a few minutes healing visualisation now and then throughout such days, but don't attempt to do too much. Take a rest, when you really need a rest. If you don't, you will be allowing the parent in you to pressurise the child in you, trying to make it do as it is told and maybe making it feel guilty, if it does not do this. Your healer, if you have one, needs to establish an adult to adult relationship with you. You need to establish an adult relationship within yourself. Get your adult in control of your life. Adult gets the fear out of cancer.

Later on, when things are going well again, you can obviously ease off to some degree. Don't get complaisant and over confident. By this time, you should be quite used to expressing your emotions more freely and openly, in whatever way seems appropriate to you. Despite this, you would be wise to go on spending some time – every day for the rest of your life – practising some healing visualisation and meditation; they should become part of your life. There are those who would argue that this will merely keep reminding you that you have had cancer and that you should forget that you have had cancer and just get on and enjoy your life. The visualisation and meditation are to remind you that your mind does control your body and that you should always consciously use your mind to keep yourself de-stressed and healthy. If that happens to remind you that you have had cancer, so be it. It is a small price to pay and it need in no way prevent you from enjoying your life. The visualisation and meditation should become an automatic part of your life, just as assertiveness and de-stressing yourself and keeping your body cleansed and well nourished, should become a part of your life, because they prove to you that you do lead a much less stressful and much more enjoyable life when you practise them all regularly. You will have moved from believing that you can heal yourself to knowing that you can heal yourself. You will have used your cancer positively, as the opportunity it can be, to change your life from the stressful experience it was, to the balanced, enjoyable, fulfilling and creative experience it should be. You will be in control of your life and in control of your health. You will have got the fear out of cancer.

Bibliography

There is a huge variety of books available on different aspects of healing. The prime message of this book is that you can learn to do all you need to do yourself, maybe with a certain amount of outside help, but even without any outside help, if you understand what you have to do and work hard at your task. I am therefore reluctant to give a long list of books for recommended reading, whilst gratefully acknowledging my debt to many authors whose books I myself have read over the years. I mention only the following few, though they all have numerous references to other books, for any who wish to read further.

The Alternative Health Guide by Brian Inglis & Ruth West, published by Mermaid Books, is a useful guide to the many alternative therapies on offer in the market place.

The Bristol Programme by Penny Brohn, published by Century, explains the holistic programme which is used at the Bristol Cancer Help Centre.

The Bristol Recipe Book by Sadhya Rippon, published by Century, explains the vegan diet used at the Bristol Cancer Help Centre and gives recipes.

Loving Medicine by Rosy Thomson MB, BCh, published by Gateway Books, gives an outline of the principles of holistic medicine and case histories from the Bristol Cancer Help Centre. The author has worked as a doctor at the Centre.

A Woman in Your Own Right by Anne Dickson, published by Quartet, is about learning to be assertive; it is for both men and women.

What Do You Say After You Say Hello by Eric Berne, published by Corgi, explains Transactional Analysis – the adult/parent/child syndrome.

Getting well again by O. Carl Simonton and Stephanie Matthews-Simonton, published by Bantam Books, explains the visualisation techniques developed in the 1970's by the Simontons with their own patients.

Cancer as a Turning Point by Lawrence LeShan PhD, published by Gateway Books, looks at some of the emotional factors in cancer. LeShan is one of the pioneers in this field.

A Cancer Therapy: Results of Fifty Cases by Dr Max Gerson M.D., published by Totality Books. This is Dr Gerson's book about his own Gerson therapy.

A Time to Heal by Beata Bishop, published by New English Library, is the story of how Beata Bishop successfully used the Gerson therapy against her cancer.